ENDURE

ENDURE

Mind, Body, and the Curiously Elastic
Limits of Human Performance

Alex Hutchinson

FOREWORD BY MALCOLM GLADWELL

wm

WILLIAM MORROW
An Imprint of HarperCollins*Publishers*

This book is for informational purposes only. Consult your health care provider before beginning any exercise plan. The author and the publisher expressly disclaim responsibility for any adverse effects arising from the use or application of the information contained herein.

HarperCollins books may be purchased for educational, business, or sales promotional use. For information, please email the Special Markets Department at SPsales@harpercollins.com.

FIRST EDITION

Library of Congress Cataloging-in-Publication Data

Names: Hutchinson, Alex, author.
Title: Endure : mind, body, and the curiously elastic limits of human
   performance / Alex Hutchinson.
Description: First edition. | New York, NY : William Morrow, 2018.
Identifiers: LCCN 2017035195 | ISBN 9780062499868 (hardback)
Subjects: LCSH: Sports--Physiological aspects. | BISAC: HEALTH & FITNESS /
   Exercise. | SPORTS & RECREATION / Running & Jogging. | SPORTS & RECREATION
   / Running & Jogging.
Classification: LCC RC1235 .H88 2018 | DDC 612/.044--dc23 LC record available at
   https://lccn.loc.gov/2017035195

18 19 20 21 22   RS/LSC   10 9 8 7 6 5 4 3

For my parents, Moira and Roger, whose curiosity, rigor, respect for differing perspectives, and talent for clarity remain the model I strive for in everything I write.

Contents

PART III: LIMIT BREAKERS / 207

Foreword

By Malcolm Gladwell

All distance runners have races that, in retrospect, make no sense. I have two. The first came when I was thirteen, in my first year of high school. With no more than a month of training under my belt, I ran a cross-country race in Cambridge, Ontario, against boys two years older than me. One of them was among the best distance runners for his age in the province. I can summon the memories of that race even today, forty years later. I simply attached myself to the leaders at the beginning and never let go, and ran myself to complete exhaustion, finishing a close and utterly inexplicable second. I say *inexplicable* because although I would go on to have a creditable career as a middle-distance runner on the track in high school, that race remains the only truly superb distance race I've ever run. I've underperformed at anything over 1,500 meters for the rest of my running life.

That is: with one exception. Two years ago, at the age of fifty-one, I ran a magical 5K in a small-town race in New Jersey, finishing a full minute faster than any 5K I'd entered since returning to serious running as a Master. On that summer day in New Jersey, I was suddenly my thirteen-year-old self from forty years ago in Cambridge. I dreamt big. I marveled at my running prowess. And then? Back to mediocrity again.

Like the obsessive person—and particularly obsessive *runner*—that I am, I have puzzled endlessly over two those anomalous races. I have running logs from my teenage years, and I've gone back over them, looking for clues. Was there some indication in my earliest training of that kind of performance? Did I do something special? For my latter 5K, of course, I have infinitely more. Months of data from Garmin on every workout leading up to the event, and then still more from the day of the race itself: pace, cadence, splits. On more than one occasion, leading up to a race, I've attempted to replicate the exact preparation I had for my New Jersey PR. I want lightning to strike twice. It hasn't, and I'm beginning to suspect the reason it hasn't is that I don't properly understand what it means to perform a feat of endurance. I think you can see where I'm going with this: I am the perfect audience for Alex Hutchinson's *Endure.*

A few words about Alex Hutchinson. We are both Canadians and both runners, although he is both a better Canadian (he still lives there; I don't) and a *much* better runner than I ever was. He invited me once to a tempo run he does with his friends on Saturday mornings in a cemetery in North Toronto. As I recall, I finished last—or maybe second last, since one of his running crew very sweetly condescended to run at my pace. Alex disappeared from sight after the first bend. As you will discover, as you continue in these pages, Alex writes about the mysteries of endurance as a student of the science, a sports fan, and a keen observer of human performance—but also as a participant. He has his own anomalous races to explain.

It must be stressed, though, that this is *not* a running book. There are plenty of running books out there, and as a runner I have read many of them. But they are insider's accounts written for other insiders: whether or not a runner should fore-foot or heel-strike, or aim for a cadence of 180 strides per minute, is a question only of significance to runners whose self-involvement extends all the way to the soles of their feet. But one of the (many) pleasures of *Endure* is how convincingly Hutchinson broadens the stakes. In one of my favorite passages, from the chapter on pain, Hutchinson writes of the attempt by Jens Voigt to break cycling's "one-hour" record. Voigt was famously indifferent to pain. But when he climbed off his bike, after breaking the record, Hutchinson tells us he was in agony: "the pain he'd been pushing to the margins of his consciousness came crashing down." That is a cycling story. But in Hutchinson's hands it also becomes a way of asking a much deeper and more consequential question about how our physiology interacts with our psychology. In a wide variety of human activity, achievement is not possible without discomfort. So what is our *relationship* to that pain? How do the signals of protest from our brain interact with the physical will to keep moving? You don't have to be a maniacal cyclist to appreciate that discussion. If anything, that discussion is likely to dissuade you from ever becoming a maniacal cyclist. "Everything was aching," Voigt said. "My neck ached from holding my head low in that aerodynamic position. My elbows hurt from holding my upper body in that position. My lungs hurt after burning and screaming for oxygen for so long. My heart hurt from the constant pounding. My back was on fire, and then there was my butt! I was really and truly in a world of pain." Oh man. It was painful just to read that passage.

Does *Endure* solve the puzzle of the anomalous race? In one sense, yes. My problem, I now realize, is that I tried to make sense of those performances using an absurdly simple model of endurance. The time I ran was my output. And so I worked backward and tried to identify the corresponding inputs that must have made it possible. Did I take one day of rest beforehand, or two? How quick was that hill workout the week before? Is there something to be learned from the last set of intervals I did? The data that we gather from our GPS sports watches makes this kind of thinking even more seductive: it encourages us to paint a simple picture of how and why our body moves through the world. After you've read *Endure*, I promise you, you'll never settle for the simple picture again. There are many things Garmin cannot tell you. And luckily, for those many things, we have Alex Hutchinson.

ENDURE

Two Hours

May 6, 2017

The broadcast booth at the Autodromo Nazionale Monza, a historic Formula One racetrack nestled in the woodlands of a former royal park northeast of Milan, Italy, is a small concrete island suspended in the air over the roadway. From this rarefied vantage point, I'm trying to offer thoughtful guest commentary to a live-streaming audience of an estimated 13 million people around the world, many of whom have roused themselves out of bed in the middle of the night to watch. But I'm getting antsy.

The race beneath me is hurtling toward a conclusion that almost no one, through months of speculation and spirited debate, had considered possible. Eliud Kipchoge, the reigning Olympic marathon champion, has been circling the racetrack for an hour and forty minutes behind an exquisitely choreographed formation of runners blocking the wind for him—and, remarkably, he's still on pace to run under two hours for 26.2 miles. Given that the world marathon record is 2:02:57, and given that records are usually shaved down in hard-fought seconds, Kipchoge's performance is already straining the limits of my ability to convey surprise and awe. Giant screens in front of me are flashing detailed statistics about Kipchoge's run, but my mind is drifting away from punditry. I want to slip out of the booth and get back down to the side of the track—to feel the crackling tension in the assembled crowd, to hear the rasp of Kipchoge's breath as he runs past, and to look into his eyes as he pushes deeper into the unknown.

———

In 1991, Michael Joyner, an ex-collegiate runner from the University of Arizona who was completing a medical residency at the Mayo Clinic in Minnesota, proposed a provocative thought experiment. The limits of endurance running, according to physiologists, could be quantified with three parameters: aerobic capacity, also known as VO_2max, which is analogous to the size of a car's engine; running economy, which is an efficiency measure like gas mileage; and lactate threshold, which dictates how much of your engine's power you can sustain for long periods of time. Researchers had measured these quantities in many elite runners, who tended to have very good values in all three parameters and exceptional values in one or two. What would happen, Joyner wondered, if a single runner happened to have exceptional—but humanly possible—values in all three parameters? His calculations suggested that this runner would be able to complete a marathon in 1:57:58.

The reactions to his paper, which was published in the *Journal of Applied Physiology*, were mostly quizzical. "A lot of people scratched their heads," Joyner recalls. The world record at the time, after all, was 2:06:50, which the Ethiopian runner Belayneh Densimo had run in 1988. A sub-two-hour marathon was not on anyone's radar—in fact, when Joyner first presented his ideas in the mid-1980s, the idea was considered so preposterous that his paper was initially rejected for publication. But the seemingly outrageous time was not a *prediction*, Joyner emphasized—it was a challenge to his fellow scientists. In some ways, his calculation was the apotheosis of a century's worth of attempts to quantify the outer limits of human endurance. This is how fast a human can run, the equations said. So what explained the chasm between theory and reality? Was it simply a question of waiting for the perfect runner to be born or the perfect race to be run—or was something missing from our understanding of endurance?

Time passed. In 1999, the Moroccan runner Khalid Khannouchi became the first person to dip below 2:06. Four years later, Paul Tergat of Kenya breached 2:05; five years after that Haile Gebrselassie of Ethiopia broke 2:04. By 2011, when Joyner and two colleagues published an updated paper in the *Journal of Applied Physiology* titled "The Two-Hour Marathon: Who and When?" the idea no longer seemed ridiculous. In fact, the journal published an unprecedented thirty-eight responses from other researchers, speculating on the various factors that might bring the barrier closer. In late 2014, shortly after Dennis Kimetto of Kenya posted the first sub-2:03, a consortium led by a British sports scientist named Yannis Pitsiladis announced plans to break the two-hour barrier within five years.

Still, two minutes and fifty-seven seconds remained a substantial gap. Also in 2014, *Runner's World* magazine asked me to undertake a comprehensive analysis of the physiological, psychological, and environmental factors that would need to come together for someone to run a two-hour marathon. After reviewing mountains of data and consulting experts around the world, including Joyner, I presented ten pages of charts, graphs, maps, and arguments, concluding with my own prediction: the barrier would fall, I wrote, in 2075.

That prediction leapt immediately to mind in October 2016, when I got an unexpected call from David Willey, then the editor in chief of *Runner's World*. Nike, the biggest sports brand in the world, was preparing to unveil a "top-secret" project that aimed to deliver a sub-two marathon in just six months. We were being offered the opportunity to go behind the scenes to cover the initiative, which they'd dubbed Breaking2. I didn't know whether to laugh or roll my eyes, but I couldn't say no. I agreed to fly to Nike's headquarters, in the Portland, Oregon, suburb of Beaverton, a few weeks later to hear their pitch. If someone had to debunk an overhyped marketing exercise, I figured the research for my earlier *Runner's World* piece had left me as well equipped as anyone.

As my guest spot on the television broadcast wraps up, Kipchoge hits twenty-three miles. It's May 6, 2017, exactly sixty-three years to the day after Roger Bannister ran the first sub-four-minute mile. I'm nearly frantic to get track-side now—but I'm not sure how to get down from my lofty perch in the broadcast booth. Peering over the edge, I briefly contemplate swinging myself over the railing and risking the drop. But a stern glance from a nearby security guard dissuades me. Instead, I head back over the causeway that connects the broadcast booth to the main building's multistory maze of dead-end hallways and unlabeled doors. I don't have time to wait for a guide. I break into a run.

Part I

MIND AND MUSCLE

CHAPTER 1

The Unforgiving Minute

If you can fill the unforgiving minute
With sixty seconds' worth of distance run,
Yours is the Earth and everything that's in it. . . .
—RUDYARD KIPLING

On a frigid Saturday night in the university town of Sherbrooke, Quebec, in February 1996, I was pondering—yet again—one of the great enigmas of endurance: John Landy. The stocky Australian is one of the most famous bridesmaids in sport, the second man in history to run a sub-four-minute mile. In the spring of 1954, after years of concerted effort, centuries of timed races, millennia of evolution, Roger Bannister beat him to it by just forty-six days. The enduring image of Landy, immortalized in countless posters and a larger-than-life bronze statue in Vancouver, British Columbia, comes from later that summer, at the Empire Games, when the world's only four-minute milers clashed head-to-head for the first and only time. Having led the entire race, Landy glanced over his left shoulder as he entered the final straightaway—just as Bannister edged past on his right. That split-second tableau of defeat confirmed him as, in the words of a British newspaper headline, the quintessential "nearly man."

But Landy's enigma isn't that he wasn't quite good enough. It's that he clearly was. In pursuit of the record, he had run 4:02 on six different occasions, and eventually declared, "Frankly, I think the four-minute mile is beyond my capabilities. Two seconds may not sound much, but to me it's like trying to break through a brick wall." Then, less than two months after Bannister blazed the trail, Landy ran 3:57.9 (his official mark in the record books is 3:58.0, since times were rounded to the nearest fifth of a second in that era), cleaving almost four seconds off his previous best and finishing 15 yards ahead of four-minute pace—a puzzlingly rapid, and bittersweet, transformation.

Like many milers before me and since, I was a Bannister disciple, with a creased and nearly memorized copy of his autobiography in permanent residence on my bedside table; but in that winter of 1996 I was seeing more and more Landy when I looked in the mirror. Since the age of fifteen, I'd been pursuing my own, lesser four-minute barrier—for 1,500 meters, a race that's about 17 seconds shorter than a mile. I ran 4:02 in high school, and then, like Landy, hit a wall, running similar times again and again over the next four years. Now, as a twenty-year-old junior at McGill University, I was starting to face the possibility that I'd squeezed out every second my body had to offer. During the long bus ride from Montreal to Sherbrooke, where my teammates and I were headed for a meaningless early-season race on one of the slowest tracks in Canada, I remember staring out the window into the swirling snow and wondering if my long-sought moment of Landyesque transformation would ever arrive.

The story we'd heard, possibly apocryphal, was that the job of designing the Sherbrooke indoor track had been assigned to the university's engineering department as a student project. Tasked with calculating the optimal angles for a 200-meter track, they'd plugged in numbers corresponding to the centripetal acceleration experienced by world-class 200-meter sprinters—forgetting the key fact that some people might want to run more than one lap at a time. The result was more like a cycling velodrome than a running track, with banks so steep that even most sprinters couldn't run in the outside lanes without tumbling inward. For middle-distance runners like me, even the inside lane was ankle-breakingly awkward; races longer than a mile had to be held on the warm-up loop around the inside of the track.

To break four minutes, I would need to execute a perfectly calibrated run, pacing each lap just two-tenths of a second faster than my best time of 4:01.7. Sherbrooke, with its amusement-park track and an absence of good competition, was not the place for this supreme effort, I decided. Instead, I would run as easily as possible and save my energy for the following week. Then, in the race before mine, I watched my teammate Tambra Dunn sprint fearlessly to an enormous early lead in the women's 1,500, click off lap after metronomic lap all alone, and finish with a scorching personal best time that qualified her for the national collegiate championships. Suddenly my obsessive calculating and endless strategizing seemed ridiculous and overwrought. I was here to run a race; why not just run as hard as I could?

Reaching the "limits of endurance" is a concept that seems yawningly obvious, until you actually try to explain it. Had you asked me in 1996 what was holding me back from sub-four, I would have mumbled something about maximal heart rate, lung capacity, slow-twitch muscle fibers, lactic acid accumulation, and various other buzzwords I'd picked up from the running magazines I devoured. On closer examination, though, none of those explanations hold up. You can hit the wall with a heart rate well below max, modest lactate levels, and muscles that still twitch on demand. To their frustration, physiologists have found that the will to endure can't be reliably tied to any single physiological variable.

Part of the challenge is that endurance is a conceptual Swiss Army knife. It's what you need to finish a marathon; it's also what enables you to keep your sanity during a cross-country flight crammed into the economy cabin with a flock of angry toddlers. The use of the word *endurance* in the latter case may seem metaphorical, but the distinction between physical and psychological endurance is actually less clear-cut than it appears. Think of Ernest Shackleton's ill-fated Antarctic expedition, and the crew's two-year struggle for survival after their ship, the *Endurance,* was crushed in the ice in 1915. Was it the toddlers-on-a-plane type of endurance that enabled them to persevere, or straightforward physical fortitude? Can you have one without the other?

A suitably versatile definition that I like, borrowing from researcher Samuele Marcora, is that endurance is "the struggle to continue against a mounting desire to stop." That's actually Marcora's description of "effort" rather than endurance (a distinction we'll explore further in Chapter 4), but it captures both the physical and mental aspects of endurance. What's crucial is the need to override what your instincts are telling you to do (slow down, back off, give up), and the sense of elapsed time. Taking a punch without flinching requires self-control, but endurance implies something more sustained: holding your finger in the flame long enough to feel the heat; filling the unforgiving minute with sixty seconds' worth of distance run.

The time that elapses can be seconds, or it can be years. During the 2015 National Basketball Association playoffs, LeBron James's biggest foe was—with all due respect to Golden State defender Andre Iguodala—fatigue. He'd played 17,860 minutes in the preceding five seasons, more than 2,000 minutes ahead of anyone else in the league. In the semis, he surprisingly asked to be pulled from a game during a tense overtime period, changed his mind, drained a three-pointer followed by a running jumper with 12.8 seconds left to seal the victory, then collapsed to the floor in a widely meme-ified swoon after the buzzer. By Game 4 of the finals, he could barely move: "I gassed out," he admitted after being held scoreless in the final quarter. It's not that he was acutely out of breath; it was the steady drip of fatigue accumulating over days, weeks, and months that just as surely pushed James to the limits of his endurance.

At the opposite end of the spectrum, even the greatest sprinters in the world fight against what John Smith, the coach of former 100-meter world-record holder Maurice Greene, euphemistically calls the "Negative Acceleration Phase." The race may be over in ten seconds, but most sprinters hit their top speed after 50 to 60 meters, sustain it briefly, then start to fade. Usain Bolt's ability to stride magisterially away from his competitors at the end of a race? A testament to his endurance: he's slowing down a little less (or a little later) than everyone else. In Bolt's

9.58-second world-record race at the 2009 World Championships in Berlin, his last 20 meters was five hundredths of a second slower than the previous 20 meters, but he still extended his lead over the rest of the field.

At the same world championships, Bolt went on to set the 200-meter world record with a time of 19.19 seconds. A crucial detail: he ran the first half of the race in 9.92 seconds—an amazing time, considering the 200 starts on a curve, but still slower than his 100-meter record. It's barely perceptible, but he was pacing himself, deliberately spreading his energy out to maximize his performance over the whole distance. This is why the psychology and physiology of endurance are inextricably linked: any task lasting longer than a dozen or so seconds requires decisions, whether conscious or unconscious, on how hard to push and when. Even in repeated all-out weightlifting efforts—brief five-second pulls that you'd think would be a pure measure of muscular force—studies have found that we can't avoid pacing ourselves: your "maximum" force depends on how many reps you think you have left.

This inescapable importance of pacing is why endurance athletes are obsessed with their splits. As John L. Parker Jr. wrote in his cult running classic, *Once a Runner,* "A runner is a miser, spending the pennies of his energy with great stinginess, constantly wanting to know how much he has spent and how much longer he will be expected to pay. He wants to be broke at precisely the moment he no longer needs his coin." In my race in Sherbrooke, I knew I needed to run each 200-meter lap in just under 32 seconds in order to break four minutes, and I had spent countless training hours learning the feel of this exact pace. So it was a shock, an eye-widening physical jolt to my system, to hear the timekeeper call out, as I completed my first circuit of the track, "Twenty-seven!"

The science of how we pace ourselves turns out to be surprisingly complex (as we'll see in later chapters). You judge what's sustainable based not only on how you feel, but on how that feeling compares to how you expected to feel at that point in the race. As I started my second lap, I had to reconcile two conflicting inputs: the intellectual knowledge that I had set off at a recklessly fast pace, and the subjective sense that I felt surprisingly, exhilaratingly good. I fought off the panicked urge to slow down, and came through the second lap in 57 seconds—and still felt good. Now I knew for sure that something special was happening.

As the race proceeded, I stopped paying attention to the split times. They were so far ahead of the 4:00 schedule I'd memorized that they no longer conveyed any useful information. I simply ran, hoping to reach the finish before the gravitational pull of reality reasserted its grip on my legs. I crossed the line in 3 minutes, 52.7 seconds, a personal best by a full nine seconds. In that one race, I'd improved more than my cumulative improvement since my first season of running, five years earlier. Poring through my training logs—as I did that night, and have many times since—revealed no hint of the breakthrough to come. My workouts suggested, at most, incremental gains compared to previous years.

After the race, I debriefed with a teammate who had timed my lap splits for me. His watch told a very different story of the race. My first lap had taken 30 seconds, not 27; my second lap was 60, not 57. Perhaps the lap counter calling the splits at the finish had started his watch three seconds late; or perhaps his effort to translate on the fly from French to English for my benefit had resulted in a delay of a few seconds. Either way, he'd misled me into believing that I was running faster than I really was, while feeling unaccountably good. As a result, I'd unshackled myself from my pre-race expectations and run a race nobody could have predicted.

After Roger Bannister came the deluge—at least, that's how the story is often told. Typical of the genre is *The Winning Mind Set,* a 2006 self-help book by Jim Brault and Kevin Seaman, which uses Bannister's four-minute mile as a parable about the importance of self-belief.

"[W]ithin one year, 37 others did the same thing," they write. "In the year after that, over 300 runners ran a mile in less than four minutes." Similar larger-than-life (that is, utterly fictitious) claims are a staple in motivational seminars and across the Web: once Bannister showed the way, others suddenly brushed away their mental barriers and unlocked their true potential.

As interest in the prospects of a sub-two-hour marathon heats up, this narrative crops up frequently as evidence that the new challenge, too, is primarily psychological. Skeptics, meanwhile, assert that belief has nothing to do with it—that humans, in their current form, are simply incapable of running that fast for that long. The debate, like its predecessor six decades ago, offers a compelling real-world test bed for exploring the various theories about endurance and human limits that scientists are currently investigating. But to draw any meaningful conclusions, it's important to get the facts right. For one thing, Landy was the only other person to join the sub-four club within a year of Bannister's run, and just four others followed the next year. It wasn't until 1979, more than twenty years later, that Spanish star José Luis González became the three hundredth man to break the barrier.

And there's more to Landy's sudden breakthrough, after being stuck for so many races, than simple mind over muscle. His six near-misses all came at low-key meets in Australia where competition was sparse and weather often unfavorable. He finally embarked on the long voyage to Europe, where tracks were fast and competition plentiful, in the spring of 1954—only to discover, just three days after he arrived, that Bannister had already beaten him to the goal. In Helsinki, he had a pacer for the first time, a local runner who led the first lap and a half at a brisk pace. And more important, he had real competition: Chris Chataway, one of the two men who had paced Bannister's sub-four run, was nipping at Landy's heels until partway through the final lap. It's not hard to believe that Landy would have broken four that day even if Roger Bannister had never existed.

Still, I can't entirely dismiss the mind's role—in no small part because of what happened in the wake of my own breakthrough. In my next attempt at the distance after Sherbrooke, I ran 3:49. In the race after that, I crossed the line, as confused as I was exhilarated, in 3:44, qualifying me for that summer's Olympic Trials. In the space of three races, I'd somehow been transformed. The TV coverage of the 1996 trials is on YouTube, and as the camera lingers on me before the start of the 1,500 final (I'm lined up next to Graham Hood, the Canadian record-holder at the time), you can see that I'm still not quite sure how I got there. My eyes keep darting around in panic, as if I expect to glance down and discover that I'm still in my pajamas.

I spent a lot of time over the next decade chasing further break-throughs, with decidedly mixed results. Knowing (or believing) that your ultimate limits are all in your head doesn't make them any less real in the heat of a race. And it doesn't mean you can simply decide to change them. If anything, my head held me back as often as it pushed me forward during those years, to my frustration and befuddlement. "It should be mathematical," is how U.S. Olympic runner Ian Dobson described the struggle to understand the ups and downs of his own performances, "but it's not." I, too, kept searching for the formula— the one that would allow me to calculate, once and for all, my limits. If I knew that I had run as fast as my body was capable of, I reasoned, I'd be able to walk away from the sport with no regrets.

At twenty-eight, after an ill-timed stress fracture in my sacrum three months before the 2004 Olympic Trials, I finally decided to move on. I returned to school for a journalism degree, and then started out as a general assignment reporter with a newspaper in Ottawa. But I found myself drawn back to the same lingering questions. Why wasn't it mathematical? What held me back from breaking four for so long, and what changed when I did? I left the newspaper and started writing as a freelancer about endurance sports—not so much about who won and who lost, but about why. I dug into the scientific literature and discovered that there was a vigorous (and sometimes rancorous) ongoing debate about those very questions.

Physiologists spent most of the twentieth century on an epic quest to understand how our bodies fatigue. They cut the hind legs off frogs and jolted the severed muscles with electricity until they stopped twitching; lugged cumbersome lab equipment on expeditions to remote Andean peaks; and pushed thousands of volunteers to exhaustion on treadmills, in heat chambers, and on every drug you can think of. What emerged was a mechanistic—almost mathematical—view of human limits: like a car with a brick on its gas pedal, you go until the tank runs out of gas or the radiator boils over, then you stop.

But that's not the whole picture. With the rise of sophisticated techniques to measure and manipulate the brain, researchers are finally getting a glimpse of what's happening in our neurons and synapses when we're pushed to our limits. It turns out that, whether it's heat or cold, hunger or thirst, or muscles screaming with the supposed poison of "lactic acid," what matters in many cases is how the brain interprets these distress signals. With new understanding of the brain's role come new—and sometimes worrisome—opportunities. At its Santa Monica, California, headquarters, Red Bull has experimented with transcranial direct-current stimulation, applying a jolt of electricity through electrodes to the brains of elite triathletes and cyclists, seeking a competitive edge. The British military has funded studies of computer-based brain training protocols to enhance the endurance of its troops, with startling results. And even subliminal messages can help or hurt your endurance: a picture of a smiling face, flashed in 16-millisecond bursts, boosts cycling performance by 12 percent compared to frowning faces.

Over the past decade, I've traveled to labs in Europe, South Africa, Australia, and across North America, and spoken to hundreds of scientists, coaches, and athletes who share my obsession with decoding the mysteries of endurance. I started out with the hunch that the brain would play a bigger role than generally acknowledged. That turned out to be true, but not in the simple it's-all-in-your-head manner of self-help books. Instead, brain and body are fundamentally intertwined, and to understand what defines your limits under any particular set of circumstances, you have to consider them both together. That's what the scientists described in the following pages have been doing, and the surprising results of their research suggest to me that, when it comes to pushing our limits, we're just getting started.

CHAPTER 2

The Human Machine

After fifty-six days of hard skiing, Henry Worsley glanced down at the digital display of his GPS and stopped. "That's it," he announced with a grin, driving a ski pole into the wind-packed snow. "We've made it!" It was early evening on January 9, 2009, one hundred years to the day since British explorer Ernest Shackleton had planted a Union Jack in the name of King Edward VII at this precise location on the Antarctic plateau: 88 degrees and 23 minutes south, 162 degrees east. In 1909, it was the farthest south any human had ever traveled, just 112 miles from the South Pole. Worsley, a gruff veteran of the British Special Air Service who had long idolized Shackleton, cried "small tears of relief and joy" behind his goggles, for the first time since he was ten years old. ("My poor physical state accentuated my vulnerability," he later explained.) Then he and his companions, Will Gow and Henry Adams, unfurled their tent and fired up the kettle. It was −31 degrees Fahrenheit.

For Shackleton, 88°23' south was a bitter disappointment. Six years earlier, as a member of Robert Falcon Scott's *Discovery* expedition, he'd been part of a three-man team that set a farthest-south record of 82°17'. But he had been sent home in disgrace after Scott claimed that his physical weakness had held the others back. Shackleton returned for the 1908–09 expedition eager to vindicate himself by beating his former mentor to the pole, but his own four-man inland push was a struggle from the start. By the time Socks, the team's fourth and final Manchurian pony, disappeared into a crevasse on the Beardmore glacier six weeks into the march, they were already on reduced rations

and increasingly unlikely to reach their goal. Still, Shackleton decided
to push onward as far as possible. Finally, on January 9, he acknowledged the inevitable: "We have shot our bolt," he wrote in his diary.
"Homeward bound at last. Whatever regrets may be, we have done
our best."

To Worsley, a century later, that moment epitomized Shackleton's
worth as a leader: "The decision to turn back," he argued, "must be
one of the greatest decisions taken in the whole annals of exploration."
Worsley was a descendant of the skipper of Shackleton's ship in the
Endurance expedition; Gow was Shackleton's great-nephew by mar-
riage; and Adams was the great-grandson of Shackleton's second in
command on the 1909 trek. The three of them had decided to honor
their forebears by retracing the 820-mile route without any outside
help. They would then take care of unfinished ancestral business by
continuing the last 112 miles to the South Pole, where they would be
picked up by a Twin Otter and flown home. Shackleton, in contrast,
had to turn around and walk the 820 miles back to his base camp—
a return journey that, like most in the great age of exploration, turned
into a desperate race against death.

What were the limits that stalked Shackleton? It wasn't just beard-
freezingly cold; he and his men also climbed more than 10,000 feet
above sea level, meaning that each icy breath provided only two-thirds
as much oxygen as their bodies expected. With the early demise of
their ponies, they were man-hauling sleds that had initially weighed
as much as 500 pounds, putting continuous strain on their muscles.
Studies of modern polar travelers suggest they were burning somewhere between 6,000 and 10,000 calories per day—and doing it on
half rations. By the end of their journey, they would have consumed
close to a million calories over the course of four relentless months,
similar to the totals of the subsequent Scott expedition of 1911–12.
South African scientist Tim Noakes argues these two expeditions
were "the greatest human performances of sustained physical endurance of all time."

Shackelton's understanding of these various factors was limited. He knew that he and his men needed to eat, of course, but beyond that the inner workings of the human body remained shrouded in mystery. That was about to change, though. A few months before Shackleton's ship, the *Nimrod*, sailed toward Antarctica from the Isle of Wight in August 1907, researchers at the University of Cambridge published an account of their research on lactic acid, an apparent enemy of muscular endurance that would become intimately familiar to generations of athletes. While the modern view of lactic acid has changed dramatically in the century since then (for starters, what's found inside the body is actually lactate, a negatively charged ion, rather than lactic acid), the paper marked the beginning of a new era of investigation into human endurance—because if you understand how a machine works, you can calculate its ultimate limits.

The nineteenth-century Swedish chemist Jöns Jacob Berzelius is now best remembered for devising the modern system of chemical notation—H_2O and CO_2 and so on—but he was also the first, in 1807, to draw the connection between muscle fatigue and a recently discovered substance found in soured milk. Berzelius noticed that the muscles of hunted stags seemed to contain high levels of this "lactic" acid, and that the amount of acid depended on how close to exhaustion the animal had been driven before its death. (To be fair to Berzelius, chemists were still almost a century away from figuring out what "acids" really were. We now know that lactate from muscle and blood, once extracted from the body, combines with protons to produce lactic acid. That's what Berzelius and his successors measured, which is why they believed that it was lactic acid rather than lactate that played a role in fatigue. For the remainder of the book, we'll refer to lactate except in historical contexts.)

What the presence of lactic acid in the stags' muscles signified was unclear, given how little anyone knew about how muscles worked. At the time, Berzelius himself subscribed to the idea of a "vital force" that powered living things and existed outside the realm of ordinary chemistry. But vitalism was gradually being supplanted by "mechanism," the idea that the human body is basically a machine, albeit a highly complex one, obeying the same basic laws as pendulums and steam engines. A series of nineteenth-century experiments, often crude and sometimes bordering on comical, began to offer hints about what might power this machine. In 1865, for example, a pair of German scientists collected their own urine while hiking up the Faulhorn, an 8,000-foot peak in the Bernese Alps, then measured its nitrogen content to establish that protein alone couldn't supply all the energy needed for prolonged exertion. As such findings accumulated, they bolstered the once-heretical view that human limits are, in the end, a simple matter of chemistry and math.

These days, athletes can test their lactate levels with a quick pinprick during training sessions (and some companies now claim to be able to measure lactate in real time with sweat-analyzing adhesive patches). But even confirming the presence of lactic acid was a formidable challenge for early investigators; Berzelius, in his 1808 book, *Föreläsningar i Djurkemien* ("Lectures in Animal Chemistry"), devotes six dense pages to his recipe for chopping fresh meat, squeezing it in a strong linen bag, cooking the extruded liquid, evaporating it, and subjecting it to various chemical reactions until, having precipitated out the dissolved lead and alcohols, you're left with a "thick brown syrup, and ultimately a lacquer, having all the character of lactic acid."

Not surprisingly, subsequent attempts to follow this sort of procedure produced a jumble of ambiguous results that left everyone confused. That was still the situation in 1907, when Cambridge physiologists Frederick Hopkins and Walter Fletcher took on the problem. "[I]t is notorious," they wrote in the introduction to their paper, "that . . . there is hardly any important fact concerning the lactic acid formation in muscle which, advanced by one observer, has not been contradicted by some other." Hopkins was a meticulous experimentalist who went on to acclaim as the codiscoverer of vitamins, for which he won a Nobel Prize; Fletcher was an accomplished runner who, as a student in the 1890s, was among the first to complete the 320-meter circuit around the courtyard of Cambridge's Trinity College while its ancient clock was striking twelve—a challenge famously immortalized in the movie *Chariots of Fire* (though Fletcher reportedly cut the corners).

Hopkins and Fletcher plunged the muscles they wanted to test into cold alcohol immediately after finishing whatever tests they wished to perform. This crucial advance kept levels of lactic acid more or less constant during the subsequent processing stages, which still involved grinding up the muscle with a mortar and pestle and then measuring its acidity. Using this newly accurate technique, the two men investigated muscle fatigue by experimenting on frog legs hung in long chains of ten to fifteen pairs connected by zinc hooks. By applying electric current at one end of the chain, they could make all the legs contract at once; after two hours of intermittent contractions, the muscles would be totally exhausted and unable to produce even a feeble twitch.

The results were clear: exhausted muscles contained three times as much lactic acid as rested ones, seemingly confirming Berzelius's suspicion that it was a by-product—or perhaps even a cause—of fatigue. And there was an additional twist: the amount of lactic acid decreased when the fatigued frog muscles were stored in oxygen, but increased when they were deprived of oxygen. At last, a recognizably modern picture of how muscles fatigue was coming into focus—and from this point on, new findings started to pile up rapidly.

The importance of oxygen was confirmed the next year by Leonard Hill, a physiologist at the London Hospital Medical College, in the *British Medical Journal*. He administered pure oxygen to runners, swimmers, laborers, and horses, with seemingly astounding results. A marathon runner improved his best time over a trial distance of three-quarters of a mile by 38 seconds. A tram horse was able to climb a steep hill in two minutes and eight seconds instead of three and a half minutes, and it wasn't breathing hard at the top.

One of Hill's colleagues even accompanied a long-distance swimmer named Jabez Wolffe on his attempt to become the second person to swim across the English Channel. After more than thirteen hours of swimming, when he was about to give up, Wolffe inhaled oxygen through a long rubber tube, and was immediately rejuvenated. "The sculls had to be again taken out and used to keep the boat up with the swimmer," Hill noted; "before, he and it had been drifting with the tide." (Wolffe, despite being slathered head-to-toe with whiskey and turpentine and having olive oil rubbed on his head, had to be pulled from the water an agonizing quarter mile from the French shore due to cold. He ultimately made twenty-two attempts at the Channel crossing, all unsuccessful.)

As the mysteries of muscle contraction were gradually unraveled, an obvious question loomed: what were the ultimate limits? Nineteenth-century thinkers had debated the idea that a "law of Nature" dictated each person's greatest potential physical capacities. "[E]very living being has from its birth a limit of growth and development in all directions beyond which it cannot possibly go by any amount of forcing," Scottish physician Thomas Clouston argued in 1883. "The blacksmith's arm cannot grow beyond a certain limit. The cricketer's quickness cannot be increased beyond this inexorable point." But what was that point? It was a Cambridge protégé of Fletcher, Archibald Vivian Hill (he hated his name and was known to all as A. V.), who in the 1920s made the first credible measurements of maximal endurance.

You might think the best test of maximal endurance is fairly obvious: a race. But race performance depends on highly variable factors like pacing. You may have the greatest endurance in the world, but if you're an incurable optimist who can't resist starting out at a sprint (or a coward who always sets off at a jog), your race times will never accurately reflect what you're physically capable of.

You can strip away some of this variability by using a time-to-exhaustion test instead: How long can you run with the treadmill set at a certain speed? Or how long can you keep generating a certain power output on a stationary bike? And that is, in fact, how many research studies on endurance are now conducted. But this approach still has flaws. Most important, it depends on how motivated you are to push to your limits. It also depends on how well you slept last night, what you ate before the test, how comfortable your shoes are, and any number of other possible distractions and incentives. It's a test of your performance on that given day, not of your ultimate capacity to perform.

In 1923, Hill and his colleague Hartley Lupton, then based at the University of Manchester, published the first of a series of papers investigating what they initially called "the maximal oxygen intake"—a quantity now better known by its scientific shorthand, VO_2max. (Modern scientists call it maximal oxygen *up*take, since it's a measure of how much oxygen your muscles actually use rather than how much you breathe in.) Hill had already shared a Nobel Prize the previous year, for muscle physiology studies involving careful measurement of the heat produced by muscle contractions. He was a devoted runner—a habit shared by many of the physiologists we'll meet in subsequent chapters. For the experiments on oxygen use, in fact, he was his own best subject, reporting in the 1923 paper that he was, at thirty-five, "in fair general training owing to a daily slow run of about one mile before breakfast." He was also an enthusiastic competitor in track and cross-country races: "indeed, to tell the truth, it may well have been my struggles and failures, on track and field, and the stiffness and exhaustion that sometimes befell, which led me to ask many questions which I have attempted to answer here."

The experiments on Hill and his colleagues involved running in tight circles around an 85-meter grass loop in Hill's garden (a standard track, in comparison, is 400 meters long) with an air bag strapped to their backs connected to a breathing apparatus to measure their oxygen consumption. The faster they ran, the more oxygen they consumed—up to a point. Eventually, they reported, oxygen intake "reaches a maximum beyond which no effort can drive it." Crucially, they could still accelerate to faster speeds; however, their oxygen intake no longer followed. This plateau is your VO_2max, a pure and objective measure of endurance capacity that is, in theory, independent of motivation, weather, phase of the moon, or any other possible excuse. Hill surmised that VO_2max reflected the ultimate limits of the heart and circulatory system—a measurable constant that seemed to reveal the size of the "engine" an athlete was blessed with.

With this advance, Hill now had the means to calculate the theoretical maximum performance of any runner at any distance. At low speeds, the effort is primarily aerobic (meaning "with oxygen"), since oxygen is required for the most efficient conversion of stored food energy into a form your muscles can use. Your VO_2max reflects your aerobic limits. At higher speeds, your legs demand energy at a rate that aerobic processes can't match, so you have to draw on fast-burning anaerobic ("without oxygen") energy sources. The problem, as Hopkins and Fletcher had shown in 1907, is that muscles contracting without oxygen generate lactic acid. Your muscles' ability to tolerate high levels of lactic acid—what we would now call anaerobic capacity—is the other key determinant of endurance, Hill concluded, particularly in events lasting less than about ten minutes.

In his twenties, Hill reported, he had run best times of 53 seconds for the quarter mile, 2:03 for the half mile, 4:45 for the mile, and 10:30 for two miles—creditable times for the era, though, he modestly emphasized, not "first-class." (Or rather, in keeping with scientific practice at the time, these feats were attributed to an anonymous subject known as "H.," who happened to be the same age and speed as Hill.) The exhaustive tests in his back garden showed that his VO_2max was 4.0 liters of oxygen per minute, and his lactic acid tolerance would allow him to accumulate a further "oxygen debt" of about 10 liters. Using these numbers, along with measurements of his running efficiency, he could plot a graph that predicted his best race times with surprising accuracy.

Hill shared these results enthusiastically. "Our bodies are machines, whose energy expenditures may be closely measured," he declared in a 1926 *Scientific American* article titled "The Scientific Study of Athletics." He published an analysis of world records in running, swimming, cycling, rowing, and skating, at distances ranging from 100 yards to 100 miles. For the shortest sprints, the shape of the world record curve was apparently dictated by "muscle viscosity," which Hill studied during a stint at Cornell University by strapping a dull, magnetized hacksaw blade around the chest of a sprinter who then ran past a series of coiled-wire electromagnets—a remarkable early system for precision electric timing. At longer distances, lactic acid and then VO$_2$max bent the world-record curve just as predicted.

But there was a mystery at the longest distances. Hill's calculations suggested that if the speed was slow enough, your heart and lungs should be able to deliver enough oxygen to your muscles to keep them fully aerobic. There should be a pace, in other words, that you could sustain pretty much indefinitely. Instead, the data showed a steady decline: the 100-mile running record was substantially slower than the 50-mile record, which in turn was slower than the 25-mile record. "Consideration merely of oxygen intake and oxygen debt will not suffice to explain the continued fall of the curve," Hill acknowledged. He penciled in a dashed near-horizontal line showing where he thought the ultra-distance records ought to be, and concluded that the longer records were weaker primarily because "the greatest athletes have confined themselves to distances not greater than 10 miles."

By the time Henry Worsley and his companions finally reached the South Pole in 2009, they had skied 920 miles towing sleds that initially weighed 300 pounds. Entering the final week, Worsley knew that his margin of error had all but evaporated. At forty-eight, he was a decade older than either Adams or Gow, and by the end of each day's ski he was struggling to keep up with them. On New Year's Day, with 125 miles still to go, he turned down Adams's offer to take some weight off his sled. Instead, he buried his emergency backup rations in the snow—a calculated risk in exchange for a savings of eighteen pounds. "Soon I was finding each hour a worrying struggle, and was starting to become very conscious of my weakening condition," he recalled. He began to lag behind and arrive at camp ten to fifteen minutes after the others.

On the eve of their final push to the pole, Worsley took a solitary walk outside the tent, as he'd done every evening throughout the trip before crawling into his sleeping bag. Over the course of the journey, he had sometimes spent these quiet moments contemplating the jagged glaciers they had just traversed and distant mountains still to come; other times, the view was simply "a never-ending expanse of nothingness." On this final night, he was greeted by a spectacular display in the polar twilight: the sun was shaped like a diamond, surrounded by an incandescent circle of white-hot light and flanked on either side by matching "sun dogs," an effect created when the sun's rays are refracted by a haze of prism-shaped ice crystals. It was the first clear display of sun dogs during the entire journey. Surely, Worsley told himself, this was an omen—a sign from the Antarctic that it was finally releasing its grip on him.

The next day was anticlimactic, a leisurely five-mile coda to their epic trip before entering the warm embrace of the Amundsen-Scott South Pole Station. They had done it, and Worsley was flooded with a sense of relief and accomplishment. The Antarctic, though, was not yet finished with him after all. Worsley had spent three decades in the British Army, including tours in the Balkans and Afghanistan with the elite Special Air Service (SAS), the equivalent of America's SEALs or Delta Force. He rode a Harley, taught needlepoint to prison inmates, and had faced a stone-throwing mob in Bosnia. The polar voyage, though, had captivated him: it demanded every ounce of his reserves, and in doing so it expanded his conception of what he was capable of. In challenging the limits of his own endurance, he had finally found a worthy adversary. Worsley was hooked.

Three years later, in late 2011, Worsley returned to the Antarctic for a centenary reenactment of Robert Falcon Scott and Roald Amundsen's race to the South Pole. Amundsen's team, skiing along an eastern route with 52 dogs that hauled sleds and eventually served as food, famously reached the Pole on December 14, 1911. Scott's team, struggling over the longer route that Shackleton had blazed, with malfunctioning mechanical sleds and Manchurian ponies that couldn't handle the ice and cold, reached it thirty-four days later only to find Amundsen's tent along with a polite note ("As you probably are the first to reach this area after us, I will ask you kindly to forward this letter to King Haakon VII. If you can use any of the articles left in the tent please do not hesitate to do so. The sledge left outside may be of use to you. With kind regards I wish you a safe return . . .") awaiting them. While Amundsen's return journey was uneventful, Scott's harrowing ordeal showed just what was at stake. A combination of bad weather, bad luck, and shoddy equipment, combined with a botched "scientific" calculation of their calorie needs, left Scott and his men too weak to make it back. Starving and frostbitten, they lay in their tent for ten snowy days, unable to cover the final eleven miles to their food depot, before dying.

A century later, Worsley led a team of six soldiers along Amundsen's route, becoming the first man to complete both classic routes to the pole. Still, he wasn't done. In 2015, he returned for yet another centenary reenactment, this time of the Imperial Trans-Antarctic Expedition—Shackleton's most famous (and most brutally demanding) voyage of all.

In 1909, Shackleton's prudent decision to turn back short of the pole had undoubtedly saved him and his men, but it was still a perilously close call. Their ship had been instructed to wait until March 1; Shackleton and one other man reached a nearby point late on February 28 and lit a wooden weather station on fire to get the ship's attention and signal for rescue. In the years after this brush with disaster, and with Amundsen having claimed the South Pole bragging rights in 1911, Shackleton at first resolved not to return to the southern continent at all. But, like Worsley, he couldn't stay away.

Shackleton's new plan was to make the first complete crossing of the Antarctic continent, from the Weddell Sea near South America to the Ross Sea near New Zealand. En route to the start, his ship, the *Endurance,* was seized by the ice of the Weddell Sea, forcing Shackleton and his men to spend the winter of 1915 on the frozen expanse. The ship was eventually crushed by shifting ice, forcing the men to embark on a now-legendary odyssey that climaxed with Shackleton leading an 800-mile crossing over some of the roughest seas on earth—in an open lifeboat!—to rugged South Georgia Island, where there was a tiny whaling station from which they could call for rescue. The navigator behind this remarkable feat: Frank Worsley, Henry Worsley's forebear and the origin of his obsession. While the original expedition failed to achieve any of its goals, the three-year saga ended up providing one of the most gripping tales of endurance from the great age of exploration—Edmund Hillary, conqueror of Mount Everest, called it "the greatest survival story of all time"—and again earned Shackleton praise for bringing his men home safely. (Three men did die on the other half of the expedition, laying in supplies at the trek's planned finishing point.)

Once more, Worsley decided to complete his hero's unfinished business. But this would be different. His previous polar treks had covered only half the actual distance, since he had flown home from the South Pole both times. Completing the full journey wouldn't just add more distance and weight to haul; it would also make it correspondingly harder to judge the fine line between stubborn persistence and recklessness. In 1909, Shackleton had turned back not because he couldn't reach the pole, but because he feared he and his men wouldn't make it back home. In 1912, Scott had chosen to push on and paid the ultimate price. This time, Worsley resolved to complete the entire 1,100-mile continental crossing—and to do it alone, unsupported, unpowered, hauling all his gear behind him. On November 13, he set off on skis from the southern tip of Berkner Island, 100 miles off the Antarctic coast, towing a 330-pound sled across the frozen sea.

That night, in the daily audio diary he uploaded to the Web throughout the trip, he described the sounds he had become so familiar with on his previous expeditions: "The squeak of the ski poles gliding into the snow, the thud of the sledge over each bump, and the swish of the skis sliding along . . . And then, when you stop, the unbelievable silence."

At first, A. V. Hill's attempts to calculate the limits of human performance were met with bemusement. In 1924, he traveled to Philadelphia to give a lecture at the Franklin Institute on "The Mechanism of Muscle." "At the end," he later recalled, "I was asked, rather indignantly, by an elderly gentleman, what use I supposed all these investigations were which I had been describing." Hill first tried to explain the practical benefits that might follow from studying athletes but soon decided that honesty was the best policy: "To tell you the truth," he admitted, "we don't do it because it is useful but because it's amusing." That was the headline in the newspaper the next day: "Scientist Does It Because It's Amusing."

In reality, the practical and commercial value of Hill's work was obvious right from the start. His VO_2max studies were funded by Britain's Industrial Fatigue Research Board, which also employed his two coauthors. What better way to squeeze the maximum productivity from workers than by calculating their physical limits and figuring out how to extend them? Other labs around the world soon began pursuing similar goals. The Harvard Fatigue Laboratory, for example, was established in 1927 to focus on "industrial hygiene," with the aim of studying the various causes and manifestations of fatigue "to determine their interrelatedness and the effect upon work." The Harvard lab went on to produce some of the most famous and groundbreaking studies of record-setting athletes, but its primary mission of enhancing workplace productivity was signaled by its location—in the basement of the Harvard Business School.

Citing Hill's research as his inspiration, the head of the Harvard lab, David Bruce Dill, figured that understanding what made top athletes unique would shed light on the more modest limits faced by everyone else. "Secret of Clarence DeMar's Endurance Discovered in the Fatigue Laboratory," the *Harvard Crimson* announced in 1930, reporting on a study in which two dozen volunteers had run on a treadmill for twenty minutes before having the chemical composition of their blood analyzed. By the end of the test, DeMar, a seven-time Boston Marathon champion, had produced almost no lactic acid—

a substance that, according to Dill's view at the time, "leaks out into the blood, producing or tending to produce exhaustion." In later studies, Dill and his colleagues tested the effects of diet on blood sugar levels in Harvard football players before, during, and after games; and studied runners like Glenn Cunningham and Don Lash, the reigning world record holders at one mile and two miles, reporting their remarkable oxygen processing capacities in a paper titled "New Records in Human Power."

Are such insights about endurance on the track or the gridiron really applicable to endurance in the workplace? Dill and his colleagues certainly thought so. They drew an explicit link between the biochemical "steady state" of athletes like DeMar, who could run at an impressive clip for extended periods of time without obvious signs of fatigue, and the capacity of well-trained workers to put in long hours under stressful conditions without a decline in performance.

At the time, labor experts were debating two conflicting views of fatigue in the workplace. As MIT historian Robin Scheffler recounts, efficiency gurus like Frederick Winslow Taylor argued that the only true limits on the productive power of workers were inefficiency and lack of will—the toddlers-on-a-plane kind of endurance. Labor reformers, meanwhile, insisted that the human body, like an engine, could produce only a certain amount of work before requiring a break (like, say, a weekend). The experimental results emerging from the Harvard Fatigue Lab offered a middle ground, acknowledging the physiological reality of fatigue but suggesting it could be avoided if workers stayed in "physicochemical" equilibrium—the equivalent of DeMar's ability to run without accumulating excessive lactic acid.

Dill tested these ideas in various extreme environments, studying oxygen-starved Chilean miners at 20,000 feet above sea level and jungle heat in the Panama Canal Zone. Most famously, he and his colleagues studied laborers working on the Hoover Dam, a Great Depression–era megaproject employing thousands of men in the Mojave Desert. During the first year of construction, in 1931, thirteen workers died of heat exhaustion. When Dill and his colleagues arrived the following year, they tested the workers before and after grueling eight-hour shifts in the heat, showing that their levels of sodium and other electrolytes were depleted—a telling departure from physico-chemical equilibrium. The fix: one of Dill's colleagues persuaded the company doctor to amend a sign in the dining hall that said THE SURGEON SAYS DRINK PLENTY OF WATER, adding AND PUT PLENTY OF SALT ON YOUR FOOD. No more men died of heat exhaustion during the subsequent four years of construction, and the widely publicized results helped enshrine the importance of salt in fighting heat and dehydration—even though, as Dill repeatedly insisted in later years, the biggest difference from 1931 to 1932 was moving the men's living quarters from encampments on the sweltering canyon floor to air-conditioned dormitories on the plateau.

If there was any remaining doubt about Hill's vision of the "human machine," the arrival of World War II in 1939 helped to erase it. As Allied soldiers, sailors, and airmen headed into battle around the world, scientists at Harvard and elsewhere studied the effects of heat, humidity, dehydration, starvation, altitude, and other stressors on their performance, and searched for practical ways of boosting endurance under these conditions. To assess subtle changes in physical capacity, researchers needed an objective measure of endurance—and Hill's concept of VO_2max fit the bill.

The most notorious of these wartime studies, at the University of Minnesota's Laboratory of Physical Hygiene, involved thirty-six conscientious objectors—men who had refused on principle to serve in the armed forces but had volunteered instead for a grueling experiment. Led by Ancel Keys, the influential researcher who had developed the K-ration for soldiers and who went on to propose a link between dietary fat and heart disease, the Minnesota Starvation Study put the volunteers through six months of "semi-starvation," eating on average 1,570 calories in two meals each day while working for 15 hours and walking 22 miles per week.

In previous VO_2max studies, scientists had trusted that they could simply ask their subjects to run to exhaustion in order to produce maximal values. But with men who've been through the physical and psychological torment of months of starvation, "there is good reason for not trusting the subject's willingness to push himself to the point at which a maximal oxygen intake is elicited," Keys's colleague Henry Longstreet Taylor drily noted. Taylor and two other scientists took on the task of developing a test protocol that "would eliminate both motivation and skill as limiting factors" in objectively assessing endurance. They settled on a treadmill test in which the grade got progressively steeper, with carefully controlled warm-up duration and room temperature. When subjects were tested and retested, even a year later, their results were remarkably stable: your VO_2max was your VO_2max, regardless of how you felt that day or whether you were giving your absolute best. Taylor's description of this protocol, published in 1955, marked the real start of the VO_2max era.

By the 1960s, growing faith in the scientific measurement of endurance led to a subtle reversal: instead of testing great athletes to learn about their physiology, scientists were using physiological testing to predict who could be a great athlete. South African researcher Cyril Wyndham argued that "men must have certain minimum physiological requirements if they are to reach, say, an Olympic final." Rather than sending South African runners all the way across the world only to come up short, he suggested, they should first be tested in the lab so that "conclusions can be drawn on the question of whether the Republic's top athletes have sufficient 'horse-power' to compete with the world's best."

In some ways, the man-as-machine view had now been pushed far beyond what Hill initially envisioned. "There is, of course, much more in athletics than sheer chemistry," Hill had cheerfully acknowledged, noting the importance of "moral" factors—"those qualities of resolution and experience which enable one individual to 'run himself out' to a far greater degree of exhaustion than another." But the urge to focus on the quantifiable at the expense of the seemingly abstract was understandably strong. Scientists gradually fine-tuned their models of endurance by incorporating other physiological traits like economy and "fractional utilization" along with VO$_2$max—the equivalent of considering a car's fuel economy and the size of its gas tank in addition to its raw horsepower.

It was in this context that Michael Joyner proposed his now-famous 1991 thought experiment on the fastest possible marathon. As a restless undergraduate in the late 1970s, Joyner had been on the verge of dropping out of the University of Arizona—at six-foot-five, and with physical endurance that eventually enabled him to run a 2:25 marathon, he figured he might make a pretty good firefighter—when he was outkicked at the end of a 10K race by a grad student from the school's Exercise and Sport Science Laboratory. After the race, the student convinced Joyner to volunteer as a guinea pig in one of the lab's ongoing experiments, a classic study that ended up demonstrating that lactate threshold, the fastest speed you can maintain without triggering a dramatic rise in blood lactate levels, is a remarkably accurate predictor of marathon time. The seed was planted and Joyner was soon volunteering at the lab and embarking on the first stages of an unexpected new career trajectory that eventually led to a position as physician-researcher at the Mayo Clinic, where he is now one of the world's mostly widely cited experts on the limits of human performance.

That first study on lactate threshold offered Joyner a glimpse of physiology's predictive power. The fact that such an arcane lab test could pick the winner, or at least the general gist of finishing order, among a group of endurance athletes was a tantalizing prospect. And when, a decade later, Joyner finally pushed this train of thought to its logical extreme, he arrived at a very specific number: 1:57:58. It was a ridiculous, laughable number—a provocation. Either the genetics needed to produce such a performance were exceedingly rare, he wrote in the paper's conclusions, "or our level of knowledge about the determinants of human performance is inadequate."

By Day 56, the relentless physical demands of Henry Worsley's solo trans-Antarctic trek were taking a toll. He woke that morning feeling weaker than he'd felt at any point in the expedition, his strength sapped by a restless night repeatedly interrupted by a "bad stomach." He set off as usual, but gave up after an hour and slept for the rest of the day. "You have to listen to your body sometimes," he admitted in his audio diary.

Still, he was more than 200 miles from his destination and already behind his planned schedule. So he roused himself that night, packed up his tent, and set off again at ten minutes after midnight under the unblinking polar sun. He was approaching the high point of the journey, slogging up a massive ice ridge known as the Titan Dome, more than 10,000 feet above sea level. The thin air forced him to take frequent breaks to catch his breath, and a stretch of sandy, blowing snow bogged his sled down and slowed his progress for several hours. By 4 P.M., having covered 16 miles in 16 hours, he was once again utterly spent. He had hoped to cross from the 89th degree of southern latitude—the one closest to the South Pole—into the 88th, but he was forced to stop one mile short of his goal. "There was nothing left in the tank," he reported. "I had completely run empty."

The next day was January 9, the day that Shackleton had famously turned back from his South Pole quest in 1909. "A live donkey is better than a dead lion, isn't it?" Shackleton had said to his wife when he returned to England. Worsley was camped just 34 miles from Shackleton's turnaround latitude, and he marked the anniversary with a small cigar—which he chomped with a gap-toothed grin, having lost a front tooth to a frozen energy bar a few days earlier—and a dram of Dewar's Royal Brackla Scotch whiskey, a bottle of which he had hauled across the continent.

Of the many advantages Worsley had over Shackleton, perhaps the most powerful was the Iridium satellite phone he carried in his pack, with which he could choose at any moment to call for an air evacuation. But this blessing was also a curse. In calculating his limits, Shackleton had been forced to leave a margin of error due to the impossibility of predicting how the return journey would go. Worsley's access to near-instantaneous help, on the other hand, allowed him to push much closer to the margins—to empty his tank day after day, after struggling through the snow for 12, 14, or 16 hours; to ignore his increasing weakness and 50-pound weight loss; to fight on even as the odds tilted further against him.

Eventually, it became clear that he wouldn't make it to his scheduled pickup. He'd been trying to log 16-hour days to get back on schedule, but soft snow and whiteouts combined with his continuing physical deterioration to derail him. He contemplated a shorter goal of reaching the Shackleton glacier, but even that proved out of reach. On January 21, his seventieth day of travel, he made the call. "When my hero Ernest Shackleton stood 97 [nautical] miles from the South Pole on the morning on January 9, 1909, he said he'd shot his bolt," Worsley reported in his audio diary. "Well today, I have to inform you with some sadness that I too have shot my bolt. My journey is at an end. I have run out of time, physical endurance, and the simple sheer ability to slide one ski in front of the other."

The next day, he was picked up for the six-hour flight back to Union Glacier, where logistical support for Antarctic expeditions is based, and then airlifted to the hospital in Punta Arenas, Chile, to be treated for exhaustion and dehydration. It was a disappointing end to the expedition, but Worsley appeared to have successfully followed Shackleton's advice to remain a "live donkey." In the hospital, though, the situation took an unexpected turn: Worsley was diagnosed with bacterial peritonitis, an infection of the abdominal lining, and rushed into surgery. On January 24, at the age of fifty-five, Henry Worsley died of widespread organ failure, leaving behind a wife and two children.

When avalanches claim a skier, or sharks attack a surfer, or a puff of unexpected wind dooms a wingsuit flier, it's always news. Like these other "extreme" deaths, Worsley's tragic end was reported and discussed around the world. There was a difference, though. There had been no avalanche, no large, hungry predator, no high-speed impact. He didn't freeze to death, he wasn't lost, and he still had plenty of food to eat. Though it may never be clear exactly what pushed him over the edge, he seemed, in essence, to have voluntarily driven himself to oblivion—a rarity that added a grim fascination to his demise. "In exploring the outer limits of endurance," Britain's *Guardian* newspaper asked, "did Worsley not realize he'd surpassed his own?"

In a sense, Worsley's death seemed a vindication of the mathematical view of human limits. "The machinery of the body is all of a chemical or physical kind. It will all be expressed some day in physical and chemical terms," Hill had predicted in 1927. And every machine, no matter how great, has a maximum capacity. Worsley, in trying to cross Antarctica on his own, had embarked on a mission that exceeded his body's capacity, and no amount of mental strength and tenacity could change that calculation.

But if that's true, then why is death by endurance so rare? Why don't Olympic marathoners and Channel swimmers and Appalachian Trail hikers keel over on a regular basis? That's the riddle a young South African doctor named Tim Noakes posed to himself as he was preparing to deliver the most important talk of his life, a prestigious honorary lecture at the annual meeting of the American College of Sports Medicine, in 1996: "I said, now hold on. What is really interesting about exercise is not that people die of, say, heatstroke; or when people are climbing Everest, it's not that one or two die," he later recalled. "The fact is, the majority don't die—and that is much more interesting."

CHAPTER 3

The Central Governor

To catch the ferry, Diane Van Deren needed to cover 36 miles in just over 8 hours. That would normally be no problem for the veteran ultra-runner—except, in this case, for the unforgiving terrain, the torrential rain and sumo-force winds left in the wake of Tropical Storm Beryl, and the fatigue and horrendous blisters accrued over the first 19 days and 900 miles of the Mountains-to-Sea Trail across North Carolina. Worse, Van Deren was startled to hear a "savage and malicious" roar from the darkness to her right. "What is that?" she yelled to her trail guide, Chuck Millsaps, the owner of a local outfitting company. It was just an airplane, he assured her—but to be safe, they strapped themselves together for mutual safety as they prepared to cross a wind-whipped bridge.

At stake in all the chaos was Van Deren's attempt to set a new record for the 1,000-mile trail: if they missed the 1 P.M. ferry from Cedar Island to Ocracoke, the mark of 24 days, 3 hours, and 50 minutes would be out of reach. The fifty-two-year-old Coloradan was a connoisseur of the slow-drip torture of ultra-endurance challenges. She had pulled a 45-pound sled 430 miles across the frozen tundra to win the Yukon Arctic Ultra (second place was—well, no other woman finished); scaled the 22,838-foot peak of Aconcagua as part of a Mayo Clinic research expedition studying human limits; and racked up top finishes at grueling races of 100 miles or more around the world. Making the ferry, though, would require squeezing a relative sprint from her battered legs. She had been running from dawn to near-dawn for almost three weeks, sleeping one to three hours a night, barely pausing to let her North Face–supported crew team duct-tape her blistered feet and cram food into her mouth.

Fortunately, Van Deren had an advantage—or at least, a unique quirk that seemed to help her push past the corporeal limits that drag down most would-be ultramarathoners. At thirty-seven, she had undergone elective brain surgery to remove a golf-ball-sized chunk of her temporal cortex, the focal point of epileptic seizures that had plagued her, as often as two or three times a week, for years. The surgery successfully stopped the seizures but also left her with neurological deficits: poor memory, an impaired sense of direction, difficulty keeping track of time. A 2011 *Runner's World* profile dubbed her "The Disoriented Express," noting that "in races she must cover hundreds of miles, and yet often has no idea how long she has been running." A significant handicap, you'd think—and yet it was only after the surgery that her racing career even started. To understand her extraordinary endurance, in other words, start with her brain.

The brain's role in endurance is, perhaps, the single most controversial topic in sports science. It's not that anyone thinks the brain doesn't matter. Everyone, right back to A. V. Hill and other pioneers of the "body as machine" view, has always understood that the race is not always to the swift—particularly if the swift make bad tactical decisions, pace themselves poorly, or simply are unwilling to suffer. In that view, the body sets the limits, and the brain dictates how close you get to those boundaries. But starting in the late 1990s, a South African physician and scientist named Tim Noakes began to argue that this picture is insufficiently radical—that it's actually the brain alone that sets and enforces the seemingly physical limits we encounter during prolonged exercise. The claim has profound and surprising implications, and the extent to which it's true or false remains one of the most volatile flashpoints in exercise physiology, two decades later.

The particular tone of the controversy has as much to do with Noakes himself—an instinctive iconoclast who has been clashing with his scientific peers more or less continuously for four decades now—as with his ideas. "Tim is probably his own worst enemy," says Carl Foster, the director of the University of Wisconsin–La Crosse's Human Performance Laboratory and a former president of the American College of Sports Medicine, who counts Noakes as a friend. "He's a very strong personality, and he gets these really neat, innovative ideas, but instead of saying, 'Wow, I've found a better way to explain this,' he says, 'Everybody else is wrong.'" (Noakes, for his part, denies ever saying that everyone else is wrong. "Of course I believe they are wrong, but I am not about to tell them that," he helpfully clarified in an email. "I just present what I believe is the truth.") Either way, Foster acknowledges, if you want to challenge a century's worth of textbook material, "maybe that stirring the pot is necessary."

Noakes started out as a collegiate rower at the University of Cape Town, but his trajectory was altered one morning in the early 1970s when his rowing practice was canceled due to high winds. His teammates went home, but Noakes decided to stay and run around a nearby lake. After forty minutes, he was overcome by a feeling of euphoria— the classic but elusive runner's high. Thanks in part to this quirk of brain chemistry, he quickly became hooked on the new sport, and ultimately shifted his professional interests from clinical medicine to running-related research. He went on to complete more than seventy marathon and ultra-marathon races, including seven finishes at South Africa's famous 56-mile Comrades Marathon.

In the lab, meanwhile, his penchant for "paradigm-rattling," as Foster calls it, emerged early. At a landmark gathering of sports scientists before the 1976 New York Marathon, at the height of the first jogging boom, most of the presentations focused on the incredible health benefits of running. Noakes, in contrast, presented the case report of an experienced marathoner who'd suffered a heart attack, puncturing the then-popular notion that marathoners were immune to clogged arteries. In 1981, he reported the case of Eleanor Sadler, a forty-six-year-old woman who collapsed during the Comrades Marathon, and diagnosed her problem as hyponatremia, a result of drinking too much, rather than the more common problem of drinking too little. It took another two decades—and a handful of deaths—before the scientific community fully acknowledged the dangers of overdrinking during exercise.

That same year, Noakes cofounded a dedicated sports science unit in the basement of the University of Cape Town's physiology department, with a single stationary bicycle and a nearly obsolete treadmill. He and his colleagues began bringing athletes in and testing their maximal oxygen consumption—"because," he says, "in 1981, to be a sports scientist, you had to have a VO_2max machine, to measure VO_2max." But it didn't take long for Noakes to grow dissatisfied with the insights provided by A. V. Hill's signature measurement. One day in the lab's early years, he tested track star Ricky Robinson and Comrades champion Isavel Roche-Kelly, less than an hour apart—and despite their vastly different racing speeds, they both recorded the same VO_2max. Noakes's conclusion: "Clearly the VO_2max was totally useless, because here we had a sub-four-minute miler and it couldn't say he was any better than the lady who could run a five-minute mile."

Over the next decade, Noakes began searching for better ways of predicting and measuring endurance, and other ways of explaining the apparent limits runners like Robinson and Roche-Kelly encountered when they finally had to step off the treadmill at the end of a test to exhaustion. Hill and his successors had focused on oxygen: at your limits, your heart was incapable of pumping any more oxygen to your muscles, or your muscles were incapable of extracting any more oxygen from your bloodstream. Noakes's first idea for an alternative to VO_2max, in the late 1980s, was that the limits might reside in the contractility of the muscle fibers themselves, but that theory fizzled.

By the 1990s, Noakes had become an internationally renowned running guru, thanks to the enduring pop-sci classic *Lore of Running*, a 944-page doorstopper that first appeared in 1985. In 1996, he received one of the highest honors in the field of exercise physiology: an invitation to deliver the J. B. Wolffe Memorial Lecture at the annual meeting of the American College of Sports Medicine. True to his reputation, he decided to harangue his eminent audience about their stubborn adherence to the "ugly and creaking edifices" of old theories that were unsupported by "empirical science." It was in preparing for this talk that he had his crucial epiphany about the rarity of deaths from exhaustion, like Henry Worsley's. Whatever our limits are, something must prevent us from exceeding them by too much. And that something, he reasoned, must be the brain.

The history of brain research is, in some ways, a tale of unfortunate injuries and illnesses. Phineas Gage, for example, was a twenty-five-year-old construction foreman working on a new railway route in 1848 when a misfired explosive blast sent a 43-inch-long tamping iron rocketing up through his cheek and out the top of his skull. His survival was remarkable enough, but even more surprising were the alterations in his personality. A polite, competent man was suddenly transformed, through damage to his frontal lobes, to a profane and unreliable one: to his friends, the doctor who treated him reported, Gage was "no longer Gage." Since then, we've learned a great deal about how the brain works by observing the distinctive changes that follow damage to different parts of the brain—an assortment of strange and mostly sad transformations of the type chronicled with tenderness and humanity by the late neurologist Oliver Sacks.

For Diane Van Deren, the first warning signs came when she was just sixteen months old, when a prolonged seizure sent her to the hospital where she lay, packed in ice, convulsing for nearly an hour. There were no apparent aftereffects, and Van Deren grew up to be a star tennis player, got married, and had children. Then, when she was twenty-nine and pregnant with her third child, the seizures returned, and over the next few years they got progressively worse. Working with neurologists at the University of Colorado, she eventually decided to have a partial right temporal lobectomy, to remove the portion of the brain where the seizures were originating. The surgery went well, and the seizures stopped—but not without a cost.

Even before the surgery, Van Deren had found running therapeutic. When she felt an "aura"—the odd out-of-body sensation that, for her, signaled an impending seizure—she was often able to ward off the seizure by heading out the door and running, sometimes for hours. After the surgery, she kept running, and began venturing farther and farther into the trails near her home south of Denver. Soon she was covering distances that would have daunted even the fittest runners, and in 2002 she entered her first ultramarathon, a 50-mile trail run with only one other entrant. The 50-miler turned out to be just a stepping-stone to 100-milers, which in turn led to multi-day races like the Yukon Arctic Ultra and, eventually, the three-week assault on the Mountains-to-Sea Trail in North Carolina in 2012.

In the final days of the record attempt, Van Deren's feet were so beat up that she had to start each day by crawling along the trail until, thanks to the familiar numbing of endorphins, she could stand up and start putting weight on them. Then she would resume clicking off the miles, one by one. By 12:20 P.M. on the twentieth day of the run, she and Millsaps were still four miles away from the crucial 1 P.M. Okracoke ferry—so they accelerated. They caught the ferry with just minutes to spare, and the ferry operator solved the mystery of the "airplane" that had buzzed them earlier: "You must have just come through those tornadoes back there," he marveled. Two days later, Van Deren climbed an 85-foot sand dune in Jockey's Ridge State Park to complete the trail in a new record of 22 days, 5 hours, and 3 minutes. "That," she told a small crowd of supporters, "is the hardest thing I have ever done."

In the *Runner's World* profile, neuropsychologist Don Gerber, who worked with Van Deren at Craig Hospital in Denver, speculated that brain surgery might have made her a better runner. Thanks to the region of her brain that was damaged, he said, "Diane's brain interprets pain differently than yours or mine does."

Van Deren, for her part, rejects this suggestion. "They all think, 'Oh, great, you don't feel pain,'" she argued in a subsequent profile.

"Well, shit—I don't feel pain? I feel pain. I just push through it." And indeed, her suffering during the run in North Carolina was evident.

Still, it's hard to escape the sense that how Van Deren experiences a prolonged endurance challenge is inescapably different from how it is for most people. Unable to read maps or keep track of where she is on a course, she doesn't focus on the challenge ahead of her. Hampered by poor short-term memory, she doesn't dwell on the effort already expended, either. "I could be out running for two weeks, but if someone told me it was day one of a race," she once joked, "I'd be like, 'Great, let's get started!'" Instead, she has no choice but to focus on the immediate task of forward motion, taking one more step, and then another. Semi-oblivious to the passage of time, she is also free of the cognitive challenge—the shackles, perhaps—of pacing herself. She is all hare and no tortoise—which, Aesopian morality aside, has its advantages.

To get a visceral feel for the struggle between mind and muscle, there's no better place to stand than at the finish line of the Comrades Marathon, the largest, oldest, and most prestigious ultra-race (that is, any race longer than the standard marathon distance of 26.2 miles) in the world, as the clock ticks down toward its rigid 12-hour cutoff. By the time the runners enter the cricket stadium in the coastal city of Durban, they've covered 56 miles of relentlessly undulating terrain, the downhills shredding their quads as mercilessly as the uphills burn their lungs, under the fierce South African sun. (In odd-numbered years, the course runs in the opposite direction, finishing in the inland city of Pietermaritzburg.)

In 2010, I joined thousands of other spectators in the stadium counting down the final seconds as the race director assumed his position on the finish line, his back to the oncoming runners and his starter's pistol pointed skyward. To be recorded as an official finisher of the race and receive a coveted finisher's medal, you have to cross the line before the 12-hour gunshot is fired. Summoning their final reserves of willpower, the runners within striking distance began to urge their battered legs into a final, frantic sprint. As the gun cracked, one man staggered across the line in 11:59:59; mere strides behind him, another man bounced off the burly course marshals who had linked arms to barricade the finish chute, while vuvuzelas sounded a mocking raspberry of defeat.

I had come to South Africa on assignment for *Outside* magazine, to write about Tim Noakes's contrarian ideas about the brain. The hook for my story was the Comrades debut of American runner Josh Cox, who was fresh off an impressive American record of 2:47:17 over 50K. I figured that if he conquered the distance, he (and Noakes, who was also in Durban to watch the race) would be able to offer vivid insights into the nature of the limits he'd had to overcome—and if the distance conquered him, the story would be even better. "The one guarantee in an event like this is the pain," Cox told me, all too prophetically, when we met for coffee the day before the race. "You have to welcome it—say 'Here you are, my friend.'" But Cox's hopes fizzled just a few miles into the race, thanks to recurring bouts of stomach cramping and diarrhea that slowed him to a walk. As familiar as this debacle might be to marathoners, these were not the limits I was hoping to write about. (The story was eventually killed.)

Still, the race had given me a perfect excuse to make a pilgrimage to one of the temples of modern exercise physiology: the next day, I flew to the opposite end of the country to spend a week visiting Noakes's lab at the University of Cape Town. At sixty, Noakes had graying temples, a near-permanent grin that expressed everything from disbelief to delight, and a habit of punctuating his sentences with the all-purpose interjection "ja." His fourth-floor office had a postcard view of Table Mountain's iconic ridgeline, and a museum's worth of sports memorabilia—framed clippings, signed rugby shirts, battered old Onitsuka Tiger running shoes—covering the walls and filling a long trophy case. On my first day there, we talked almost nonstop for four hours ("I don't normally have much lunch," he said, a bit apologetically, when I proposed a break, "but you're welcome to if you'd like") as he recounted the origins of what has become known as the "central governor" theory.

In his keynote lecture at the 1996 ACSM conference, Noakes had argued that A. V. Hill's concept of VO_2max was fundamentally flawed: that physical exhaustion isn't a consequence of the heart's inability to pump enough oxygen to the muscles. Otherwise, he reasoned, the heart itself, and perhaps the brain, would also be starved of oxygen, with catastrophic results. He liked to point out a famous picture of South African marathoner Josia Thugwane, moments after winning the 1996 Olympic marathon, jogging around the track with silver medalist Lee Bong-Ju, whom he had outsprinted by just three seconds. "Do you notice he's not dead?" he'd say, pointing at Lee. "What does that tell you? It means he could have run faster."

But if Hill's ideas about oxygen were wrong, what was the alternative? Noakes felt the brain had to be involved, and in a 1998 paper he coined the term "central governor," borrowing terminology that A. V. Hill himself had used seventy years earlier. But the details remained unclear. Over the next decade, working with collaborators such as Alan St. Clair Gibson, then at the University of Cape Town, Frank Marino, of Charles Sturt University in Australia, and a succession of other students and postdoctoral researchers in his own lab, he began to assemble a coherent picture with two key planks. First, the limits we encounter during exercise aren't a consequence of failing muscles; they're imposed in advance by the brain to ensure that we never reach true failure. And second, the brain imposes these limits by controlling how much muscle is recruited at a given effort level (an idea we'll explore in detail in Chapter 6).

The first point—the concept of "anticipatory regulation," as Noakes and his colleagues refer to it—is subtle, so it's worth pausing to unpack it. Long before Noakes, researchers had theorized that the brain might sense distress signals from elsewhere in the body and shut things down when the warnings exceeded a critical level. Exercise in the heat is a classic example: if you run to exhaustion on a treadmill in a hot room, your brain will stop driving your muscles when your core temperature hits a critical threshold of about 104 degrees Fahrenheit. But Noakes takes this idea a step further, arguing that in real-world situations like running a 10K on a hot day, the brain gets involved long before you reach that critical temperature. You don't hit 104 and keel over; you slow down and run at a pace that keeps you below 104.

The most controversial claim is that this pacing instinct isn't entirely voluntary: your brain forces you to slow down, long before you're in real physiological distress. In experiments led by Noakes's student Ross Tucker, cyclists started at a slower pace right from the outset when the temperature was high—and crucially, the amount of muscle recruited by the brain was also lower within the first few minutes. At a conscious level, the cyclists were trying just as hard (as their reported level of effort indicated), but fewer muscle fibers in their legs were contracting thanks to their central governor's inbuilt caution. The difference between the traditional and revised views of the brain's role, Tucker explained during my visit in Cape Town, is that "they're really looking at the off switch, whereas we're looking at the dimmer control."

It's easy to get lost in the weeds of this debate. Over the course of my visit, I spent hours with various students, postdocs, and colleagues of Noakes, learning about the various tentacles of evidence that buttressed their brain-centered view of endurance. There were longstanding historical anomalies, like the puzzlingly low lactate levels observed when people exercise to exhaustion at high altitudes, contrary to what Hill's model would predict. And there was a steady stream of new observations: an instant performance boost when you swish a carbohydrate drink in your mouth and then trick your brain by spitting it out; marathon runners setting world records despite supposedly crippling levels of dehydration; brain-altering drugs like Tylenol that boost endurance without any effect on the muscles or heart.

But when I asked Noakes for the single most convincing piece of evidence in favor of his theory, he said, without hesitation, "the end spurt." How could the runners at Comrades, after pushing themselves through 56 miles of hell, summon a finishing sprint to beat the 12-hour limit? Conventional physiology suggests that you get progressively more fatigued over the course of a run, as muscle fibers fail and fuel stores are emptied. But then, when the end is in sight, you speed up. Clearly your muscles were capable of going faster in the preceding miles; so why didn't they? "That shows that our understanding of fatigue is totally wrong," Noakes said. It must be the brain that holds you back during long efforts, and then releases the final reserves when you're nearly finished and the danger is past.

I always try to evaluate scientific theories dispassionately, based on evidence rather than anecdote. But in this case, my head was nodding involuntarily as Noakes spoke. This phenomenon wasn't just familiar to me—it was, in some ways, my nemesis. In my mid-twenties, after a few injury-plagued years, I'd moved up from 1,500 to 5,000 meters. But every time I raced the longer distance, my pace would gradually tail off in the later stages of the race—and then I'd launch a sizzling last lap, leaving everyone (including myself) puzzled about why I had slowed down so much in the previous laps. At first I chalked it up to inexperience, and then to lack of concentration. And there may be some truth to both those explanations, but it felt like something deeper.

By the time I ran what would turn out to be my fastest 5,000, on a perfect evening in Palo Alto, California, in 2003, I'd decided I needed a new mental strategy: I would pretend I was only running 4,000 meters, and simply not worry if I had to jog the last kilometer. I wanted to run 2:45 per kilometer, and my first three kilometers were 2:45, 2:45, 2:47. The moment of truth: I knuckled down and vowed to run the fourth kilometer as hard as I could—but little by little, I drifted back from the pack I was running with. My next split was a disappointing 2:53. That was as fast as I could move my legs, and my pace slowed even more as I entered the final kilometer. I'd bitten off more than I could chew and was paying the price.

At most track races, officials mark the start of your final 400-meter lap by ringing a cowbell in your ear. It's a handy Pavlovian cue that tells you that your suffering is almost over. And on that night on the Stanford track, I once again felt the curious and familiar transformation in my legs as the bell rang for me. I passed ten runners while running the last lap in around 57 seconds, a full 10 seconds faster than my average pace for the race. My last kilometer, at 2:42, was my fastest even though I only started sprinting with a lap to go. And—I can't emphasize this enough—I was trying as hard as I could right up to the penultimate lap. A friend who'd come to watch asked if I was trying to impress her by slowing down late in the race so I could finish with a flourish. No, I said, I just . . . But I didn't have an explanation. I didn't understand it myself.

As it turns out, it's not just me. Noakes showed me a study that he, Tucker, and Michael Lambert had published in 2006, analyzing the pacing patterns of almost every world record set in the modern era in the men's 800 meter, mile, 5,000, and 10,000 meter races. For the three longer races, the pattern was startlingly consistent: after a quick start, the record breakers would settle into a steady pace until the final stages of the race. Then, even though they were running faster than they'd ever run before, and their oxygen-starved muscles were presumably awash in a sea of fatigue-inducing metabolites, they accelerated. Of the 66 world records in the 5,000 and 10,000 meters dating back to the early 1920s, the last kilometer was either the fastest of the race or the second fastest (behind the opening kilometer) in all but one. I was willing to attribute my own uneven pacing to incompetence—but these were the finest runners in history on the best day of their lives, which suggests that the pattern is more deeply ingrained than a mere pacing error.

In fact, there's good reason to think that pacing is driven as much by instinct as by choice, according to Dominic Micklewright, a researcher at the University of Essex. Micklewright followed an unorthodox route to academia, going straight from high school to the Royal Navy, where he served as a diver on nuclear submarines for seven years, and then spending nine years as a police officer in London before studying sport and exercise psychology. His interest in pacing dates back to his training as a military diver, when he and the other

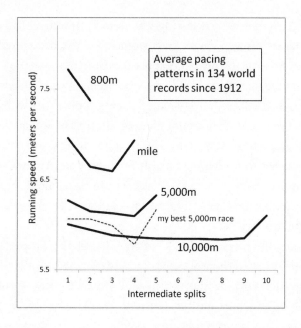

World records in long-distance races are run with a strikingly consistent pattern that includes an acceleration in the final stages, according to a 2006 analysis in the International Journal of Sports Physiology and Performance. *This finishing kick is notably absent in shorter 800-meter races, for reasons we'll discuss in Chapter 6. The intermediate splits above are every 400 meters for the two shorter races, and every 1,000 meters for the two longer ones.*

trainees had to swim submerged to the other end of a 1,200-meter saltwater lake on Horsea Island, on Britain's south coast, without using up their supply of air. "If they caught you breaching, you would get clobbered over the back of the head with an oar, or they'd throw in one of those underwater scare charges," he recalls. With that incentive, you inevitably thought very carefully about the challenge of spending your energy—and oxygen—as frugally as possible.

In 2012, Micklewright had more than a hundred schoolchildren ranging in age from five to fourteen complete a battery of tests to assess their cognitive development, in order to slot them into one of the four developmental stages proposed by Swiss psychologist Jean Piaget;

then the kids ran a race lasting about four minutes. The younger kids in the two lower Piaget stages opted for the unfettered sprint-and-then-hang-on-for-dear-life approach, starting fast then steadily fading. In contrast, the kids in the two higher Piaget stages had already adopted the familiar U-shaped pacing profile that world-record holders use: a fast start, gradual slowing, then a fast finish. Sometime around the age of eleven or twelve, in other words, our brains have already learned to anticipate our future energy needs and hold back something in reserve—a relic, Micklewright speculated, of the delicate balance between searching for food and conserving energy deep in our evolutionary past.

Not everyone buys Noakes's argument that pacing patterns like the end spurt reveal the workings of a central governor. For example, it could be that you speed up at the end of a race because you finally tap into your precious but limited reserves of anaerobic energy, the high-octane fuel source that powers you in short races lasting less than a minute. But there are other hints that the finishing kick isn't just physiological.

In 2014, a group of economists from the University of Southern California; the University of California, Berkeley; and the University of Chicago mined a massive dataset containing the finish times of more than nine million marathoners from races around the world spanning four decades. The distribution of finishing times looks a bit like the classic bell-shaped curve, but with a set of spikes superimposed. Around every significant time barrier—three hours, four hours, five hours—there are far more finishers than you'd expect just below the barrier, and fewer than you'd expect just above. Similar but smaller spikes show up at half-hour intervals, and there are barely perceptible ripples even at ten-minute increments. The cruel metabolic demands of the marathon, which inevitably depletes your stores of readily available fuel, mean that most people are slowing in the final miles. But with the right incentive, some are able to speed up—and it's only the brain that can respond to abstract incentives like breaking four hours for an arbitrary distance like 26.2 miles.

A further curious detail from this dataset: the faster the runners were, the less likely they were able to summon a finishing sprint. Of the runners finishing near the three-hour barrier, about 30 percent were able to speed up in the final 1.4 miles of the race; 35 percent of those trying to break four hours sped up; and more than 40 percent of those trying to break five hours managed it. One possible interpretation is that, over the course of their long hours of training, the more committed runners had gradually readjusted the settings on their central governors, learning to leave as little as possible in reserve. Perhaps that's another, slower way of achieving the run-in-the-present-moment strength that allows Diane Van Deren to race so close to her limits. I tried to trick myself into forgetting the last kilometer of my 5,000-meter races; Van Deren's bittersweet gift is that she can forget without even trying.

Right from the start, the central governor proposal was highly controversial. After his 1996 speech, Noakes recalls, "people got very, very angry." There were rebuttals and surrebuttals in a cycle that is still continuing, more than two decades later. In a 2008 article in the *British Journal of Sports Medicine,* Noakes argued that physiologists' focus on VO_2max had "produced a brainless model of human exercise performance." Roy Shephard, an influential professor emeritus at the University of Toronto, shot back with an article in the journal *Sports Medicine* in 2009 titled "Is It Time to Retire the 'Central Governor'?" Following a further exchange, Shephard concluded, "In the parlance of my North American colleagues, the time may now be ripe for proponents of the hypothesis to 'Put up or shut up.'"

If anything, the controversies swirling around Noakes have increased since his retirement from the University of Cape Town in 2014. His book on hydration, *Waterlogged,* accused most of the world's leading hydration researchers, including former colleagues and collaborators, of selling out to the commercial interests of sports-drink makers. He is now a vocal proponent of low-carb, high-fat diets for both health and athletic performance, leading him to disown the chapters he wrote on nutrition and carbohydrate loading in *Lore of Running* and earning him a disciplinary hearing that threatened to revoke his medical license after he tweeted advice to a breastfeeding mother about weaning babies onto a low-carb, high-fat diet.

As these other battles rage, the central governor controversy has to some extent faded into the background. With their own retirements on the horizon, it's clear that the older generation of physiologists— Noakes's peers—will never be convinced. On the other hand, says American Society of Exercise Physiologists cofounder Robert Robergs of Noakes's influence, "most of the younger breed of exercise physiologists, in which I would group myself, recognize that, boy, some of his challenges are correct." Whether the brain plays a role in defining the limits of endurance is no longer in doubt; the debate now is how.

One way to answer that question would be to peer inside the brain during strenuous exercise—a task that, until recently, was completely impossible. With advances in brain imaging, it's now just very, very difficult. Functional magnetic resonance imaging, or fMRI, allows researchers to observe changes in blood flow to different regions of the brain with great spatial precision, but can't capture changes that occur in less than a second or two. You also have to remain perfectly still inside the bore of a powerful magnet—a restriction that presents serious challenges for exercise studies. During my visit to Cape Town, Noakes showed me video of a Rube Goldberg–esque contraption, developed by collaborators in Brazil, that allows subjects to pedal an externally mounted bike (you can't have metal parts in the same room as the MRI magnet) via a 10-foot-long driveshaft, while lying supine inside the cylindrical bore of the magnet, with cushions jammed around their heads to keep them still. But the initial results, published in 2015, didn't manage to push subjects to exhaustion and produced unclear patterns of brain activity.

Other researchers have tried electroencephalography, or EEG, which uses a web of electrodes mounted on the head to measure the brain's electrical activity. The advantage of EEG is that it can truly measure changes in real time; the disadvantage is that it's highly sensitive to body or head motion—just blinking or letting your gaze wander garbles the results. Such studies are already yielding insights about the brain areas involved in fatigue, and (as we'll see in Chapter 12) even being used to identify promising regions for electrical stimulation in an attempt to enhance endurance.

But these approaches are unlikely to ever truly pinpoint the central governor. "One of the big issues with the central governor is that it was initially portrayed to be a specific point, as if there was going to be one structure that did all this," Tucker told me. "And people were like, show me the structure." But endurance isn't simply a dial in the brain; it's a complex behavior that will involve nearly every brain region, Tucker suspects, which makes proving its existence (or nonexistence) a dauntingly abstract challenge.

Ultimately, the most convincing route to proving the central governor's existence might also be the first and most obvious question that pops into people's minds when they first hear about the theory, which is: Can you change its settings? Can you gain access to at least some of the emergency reserve of energy that your brain protects? There's no doubt that some athletes are able to wring more out of their bodies than others, and those who finish with the most in reserve would dearly love to be able to reduce that margin of safety. But is this really a consequence of the brain's subconscious decision to throttle back muscle recruitment—or is it, as a rival brain-centered theory of endurance posits, simply a matter of how badly you want it?

CHAPTER 4

The Conscious Quitter

Since the days of Marco Polo, no trip along the Silk Road has ever been straightforward—and Samuele Marcora's 13,000-mile motorcycle ride from London overland to Beijing in 2013 was no exception. Unlike Polo, Marcora didn't encounter any dragons or men with dogs' faces along the route, but he and his trip-mates did spend seventeen hours crossing the Caspian Sea on a rusty Soviet-era freighter; navigate the crumbling roads and stifling bureaucracy of Turkmenistan, Uzbekistan, Tajikistan, and Kyrgyzstan (the 'Stans, as he refers to them affectionately); skid along endless soft sand and mud trails in the thin air of the Tibetan plateau, up to 16,700 feet above sea level, for two weeks; and splash through monsoon-drenched roads on the final leg of their journey through China. Oh, and he also broke his ankle in Uzbekistan and shattered a rib on the road from Everest Base Camp, making the bone-rattling corrugated roads of Central Asia even more painful than normal.

In a sense, all of these stressors were part of the plan. Their inevitability was the reason Marcora, an exercise scientist in the University of Kent's Endurance Research Group, joined the eighty-day expedition, which was organized by adventure motorcycling outfitter GlobeBusters. Packed on the back of Marcora's BMW R1200GS Triple Black was his "lab in a pannier," crammed with portable scientific equipment to perform daily measurements of the trip's mounting mental and physical toll, with himself and his thirteen fellow riders as lab rats: swallowable thermometer pills to record core temperature, "bioharness" straps to record heart rhythms and breathing rate, a finger-mounted oximeter to measure oxygen saturation in the blood, a grip-strength tester to measure muscular fatigue, a portable reaction-time device to assess cognitive fatigue, and more.

Marcora's interest in adventure motorcycling dates back to his teens. His first long trip, as a fourteen-year-old growing up in northern Italy, was a solo ride of more than 100 miles from his hometown outside Milan to Lake Maggiore, near the Swiss border, to visit his girlfriend. He taped a map to the gas tank of his 50cc Fantic Caballero dirt bike and navigated on back roads, to avoid the highways he wasn't yet allowed to drive on. But he also nurtured an interest in bikes of the nonpowered variety—and, more broadly, in the enduring riddle of endurance. He trained as an exercise physiologist, and early in his career served as a consultant for Mapei Sport Service, a research center charged with providing a scientific edge for one of the top road cycling teams in the world in the 1990s and early 2000s, publishing research on mountain biking and soccer. His focus, as for thousands of other physiologists around the world, was on figuring out how to extend the limits of the human body by a percent here and a fraction of a percent there.

It was his mother—a very important figure in any Italian man's life, he says, only half-jokingly—who gave his career trajectory a crucial nudge in a new direction. In 2001 she was diagnosed with thrombotic thrombocytopenic purpura, a rare autoimmune disorder that causes tiny blood clots to form in small blood vessels throughout the body. After one attack, she was left with kidney damage that necessitated seven years of dialysis and, eventually, a transplant. What puzzled her son was the seemingly subjective nature of the extreme fatigue that she and other patients with similar conditions endured, which fluctuated rapidly and couldn't be clearly linked to any single physical root cause—a disconnect reminiscent of other enigmatic conditions like chronic fatigue syndrome. The feeling of fatigue was debilitating, but from the usual below-the-neck perspective of an exercise physiologist, there was seemingly nothing to fix.

This riddle led Marcora to the brain—and to tackle it, he decided he needed to learn more about what brain experts already knew. In 2006, he took a sabbatical from his teaching position at the University of Bangor, in Wales, to take courses in the university's psychology department. Over the next few years, he formulated a new "psychobiological" model of endurance, integrating exercise physiology, motivational psychology, and cognitive neuroscience. In his view, the decision to speed up, slow down, or quit is always voluntary, not forced on you by the failure of your muscles. Fatigue, in other words, ultimately resides in the brain—an insight as relevant to motorcyclists as to marathoners. As Marcora rolled along the Silk Road collecting data on the mental and physical performance of his fellow adventure riders, he was gathering support for his contention that mind and muscle are inextricably linked—a brain-centered view of endurance, like Tim Noakes's central governor, but with several key differences.

In 2011, I drove 120 miles through Australia's Blue Mountains from Sydney, where I was living at the time, to an old gold-rush town in the country's sparsely populated interior called Bathurst. The local campus of Charles Sturt University was hosting an international conference called "The Future of Fatigue: Defining the Problem"—a title that reflected the continuing controversy and confusion surrounding even the most basic concepts in endurance research. "Every time I say the word 'fatigue' I have to put it in quotes," joked one of the hosts, "because I'm not even sure what it means." Scientists from around the world had gathered to present their ideas and try to hash out their differences. One of the featured speakers, and the main reason I'd decided to make the trip, was Samuele Marcora.

Marcora had made his first big splash two years earlier, not just among researchers but among the *New York Times*–reading public, with a provocative study of mental fatigue. He'd asked sixteen volunteers to complete a pair of time-to-exhaustion tests on a stationary bike. Before one of the tests, the subjects spent 90 minutes performing a mentally fatiguing computer task that involved watching a series of letters flash on a screen, and clicking different buttons as quickly as possible depending on which letters appeared. It's not a particularly difficult task, but it requires sustained focus—and doing it for 90 minutes is definitely draining. Before the other cycling test, the subjects spent the same 90 minutes watching a pair of bland documentaries ("World Class Trains—The Venice Simplon Orient Express" and "The History of Ferrari—The Definitive Story"), specifically chosen to be "emotionally neutral."

Depending on how you look at it, the results were either utterly predictable or, from the perspective of textbook physiology, inexplicable. After the mentally draining computer game, the subjects gave up 15.1 percent sooner in the cycling test, stopping on average at 10 minutes and 40 seconds compared to 12 minutes and 34 seconds. It wasn't because of any detectable physiological fatigue: heart rate, blood pressure, oxygen consumption, lactate levels, and a host of other metabolic measurements were identical during the two trials. Motivation levels, as measured by psychological questionnaires immediately before the cycling tests, were the same—helped along by a £50 prize for top performance. The only difference was that, right from the very first pedal stroke, the mentally fatigued subjects reported higher levels of perceived exertion. When their brains were tired, pedaling a bike simply felt harder.

The system Marcora used to measure perceived exertion was called the Borg Scale, named for Swedish psychologist Gunnar Borg, who pioneered its use in the 1960s. Though there are many variations, Borg's original scale ran from 6 ("no effort at all") to a maximum of 20 (the penultimate value, 19, was defined as "very, very hard"), with the numbers corresponding very roughly to your expected heart rate divided by ten. A Borg score of 13 to 14, for example, corresponds to an effort you'd call "somewhat hard," which would produce a heart rate of 130 to 140 beats per minute in most people. But Borg viewed the effort scale as far more than a convenient shortcut for researchers whose heart-rate monitor ran out of batteries. "In my opinion," he wrote, "perceived exertion is the single best indicator of the degree

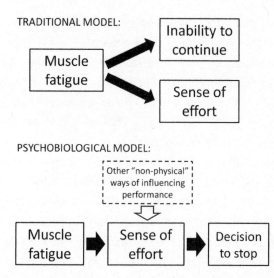

In the conventional "human machine" view of endurance (top), physical
fatigue in the muscles directly causes you to slow down or stop; how hard
the effort feels is merely an incidental by-product. In Samuele Marcora's
psychobiological model (bottom), effort is what connects physical fatigue
to performance—which means that anything that alters your perception
of effort (subliminal messages, mental fatigue, etc.) can alter your endurance, independent of what's happening in your muscles.

of physical strain," since it integrates information from muscles and
joints, the cardiovascular and respiratory systems, and the central
nervous system.

In his talk at the conference in Bathurst, Marcora took this argument a step further. Perceived exertion—what we'll refer to in this
book as your sense of effort—isn't just a proxy for what's going on in
the rest of your body, he argued. It's the final arbiter, the only thing
that matters. If the effort feels easy, you can go faster; if it feels too
hard, you stop. That may sound obvious, or even tautological, but it's a
profound statement—because, as we'll discover, there are lots of ways
you can alter your sense of effort, and thus your apparent physical
limits, without altering what's happening in your muscles. Case in

point: getting mentally fatigued increases your sense of effort (by between one and two points on the Borg scale, in Marcora's protocol) and thus reduces endurance. By definition, the cyclists always decided to quit as their perceived exertion approached the maximum of 20; they just reached that point sooner when they were mentally fatigued.

If effort is the yin of Marcora's psychobiological model, motivation is the yang. We're not always willing to push to an effort of 20, which is one reason athletes rarely produce world records or even personal bests in training. In his talk, Marcora offered a now-classic illustration of this, from a 1986 experiment by French researcher Michel Cabanac. Cabanac asked volunteers to sit bent-legged against a wall with no chair for as long as they could, offering varying rewards for each 20-second period they stayed in position. When the subjects were offered 0.2 francs per 20 seconds, their quads gave out after just over two minutes, on average; when they were offered 7.8 francs per 20 seconds, their endurance magically doubled. If the moment of collapse was dictated by a failure of the muscles, how did the muscles know about the richer payoff?

Marcora himself produced a similar mind-over-muscle demonstration with a group of elite rugby players who competed in a time-to-exhaustion cycling test. At an average target power of 242 watts, which corresponded to 80 percent of their peak power, the players lasted for about 10 minutes, with cash prizes to ensure they fully exhausted themselves. As soon as they gave up—within three to four seconds—they were asked to see how much power they could generate in a single 5-second burst of pedaling. Curiously, although they had just declared themselves incapable of producing 242 watts, they managed to average 731 watts during this five-second sprint. It follows that the subjects didn't stop the test because their muscles were physically incapable of producing the required power; instead, the researchers argued, it was perception of effort that mattered.

At the exercise physiology conference in Bathurst, Marcora laid out his case with characteristic zeal. Amid the mostly uniform crowd of tracksuit-clad ex-athletes, he cut a swashbuckling figure, with untucked shirt, permastubbled jaw, and casual asides about his plan to motorcycle along Australia's Great Ocean Road after the conference. At one point, he showed a bewilderingly complex slide taken from a recent paper describing the conventional model of endurance fatigue— a flow chart with forty-four different boxes ranging from heart rate to "mitochondrial density/enzyme activity"—and then compared it to the equations for general relativity and quantum mechanics. "Physicists can explain the whole universe with two theories, and they're not happy with that," he said. "Endurance performance is complicated, but it's not more complicated than the entire universe!"

The simple alternative, Marcora argued, is that anything that moves the "effort dial" in your head up or down affects how far or fast you can run. All the usual physical cues—dehydration, tired muscles, a pounding heart—contribute to how hard an effort feels. Athletes train their bodies to adapt to those cues, and over time the effort of running at a given pace gets lower. But less obvious factors, like mental fatigue, also contribute to how hard your run feels—and trying to hold marathon pace for hours and hours, for example, is pretty taxing on the brain. This, Marcora told the conference, leads to a radical idea: If you could train the brain to become more accustomed to mental fatigue, then—just like the body—it would adapt and the task of staying on pace would feel easier. "I have an eye for things that at a superficial level seem crazy," he said. "If I tell somebody, okay, I'm going to improve your endurance performance by making you sit in front of a computer and do things on a keyboard, you will think I'm nuts. But if something can fatigue you, and you repeat it over time systematically, you'll adapt and get better at the task. That's the basis of physical training. So my reasoning is simple: We should be able to get the same effect by using mental fatigue."

This was an unexpectedly bold prediction, so I cornered Marcora during a break after his talk to find out more. He was designing a study to test whether "brain endurance training"—weeks of doing mentally fatiguing computer tasks—could, without any change in physical training, make people faster. I pestered him for details and asked if I could try it. He patiently answered my questions, then added a warning. "People who have done these mental fatigue studies—it's not nice," he said. "It's really bad. They hate you at the end of the task."

In June 1889, as the academic term at the University of Turin drew to a close, a physiologist named Angelo Mosso conducted a series of experiments on his fellow professors before and after they administered their year-end oral exams. He attached a two-kilogram weight to a string, and asked the professors to raise and lower the weight every two seconds by flexing their middle fingers, and then repeated the task using electric shocks to force the fingers to contract. The number of contractions they managed after three and a half hours of grilling their students was dramatically reduced compared to their baseline performance—a clear indication that "intellectual labor" had sapped their muscular endurance.

Mosso's results, which were collected in an influential text called *La Fatica* ("Fatigue") in 1891, were the first scientific demonstration of the physical effects of mental fatigue. Like later fatigue researchers such as A. V. Hill and David Bruce Dill, Mosso was motivated by concerns about industrial working conditions. For Mosso, the working-class son of an impoverished carpenter, the conditions in sulfur mines and Sicilian farms, particularly for child laborers, amounted to an injustice "worse than slavery, worse than the dungeon." Just as mental fatigue sapped physical strength, he argued, physical fatigue stunted mental growth in overworked child miners, so that "those who survive become wicked, villainous, and cruel." By rigorously measuring the effects of fatigue, he hoped to encourage the passage of laws to protect the vulnerable—for instance, by limiting the workday of children between nine and eleven to at most eight hours.

Unlike Marcora's results 120 years later, Mosso's mental-fatigue studies weren't seen as particularly surprising. This was before the idea of the "human machine" had become entrenched, so the idea that physical performance might depend as much on willpower as on muscle power seemed natural. As time passed, though, Mosso's insights were mostly forgotten and discussions of the brain's role in endurance dropped out of exercise physiology textbooks. The torch passed instead to psychologists, who in the late 1800s began turning their attention to sports.

An 1898 study by Indiana University psychologist Norman Triplett, in which he explored why cyclists ride faster with others than alone, is often pegged as the debut of sports psychology as a distinct discipline. In addition to the aerodynamics of drafting—what Triplett termed the "Suction Theory" and the "Shelter Theory"—he considered psychological explanations such as "brain worry" for the link between mind and muscle, as well as the idea that heavy exercise "poisons" the blood, which in turn "benumbs the brain and diminishes its power to direct and stimulate the muscles." He even speculated that a cyclist following behind another cyclist might become hypnotized by the motion of the wheel in front of him, producing performance-enhancing "muscular exaltation." The field didn't take off immediately: the first dedicated sports psychology lab in the United States, founded in 1925 at the University of Illinois, petered out in 1932 due to a lack of interest and funding. Still, by the second half of the twentieth century, sports psychology was established as a legitimate sub-field, with its own entirely separate body of knowledge about the brain's role in endurance.

When I was in university, in the 1990s, our track team giggled through group sessions with a sports psychologist who introduced us to an arsenal of techniques meant to help us perform optimally—visualization, relaxation, and so on. We memorized a five-step self-talk technique for stopping negative thoughts that might arise during a race: Recognize, Refuse, Relax, Reframe, Resume. That's what we would yell to anyone who started to drift off the pace during a long, grueling workout. It was a joke to us. None of us actually tried to apply these techniques with any seriousness—because victory, we knew, was the straightforward result of pumping the most oxygen to the fittest muscles.

This schism between psychology and exercise physiology is what

Marcora, trained as an exercise physiologist, was hoping to address when he spent his mid-career sabbatical term studying psychology. A truly universal theory of endurance, he felt, should be able to use the same theoretical framework to explain how both mental and physical factors—self-talk and sports drinks, say—alter your performance. And in the psychobiological model that he came up with, the link between old-school sports psychology techniques and actual physiological outcomes suddenly seems much more plausible. After all, the perception of effort—the master controller of endurance, in Marcora's view—is a fundamentally psychological construct.

For example, a famous 1988 experiment conducted by psychologists at the University of Mannheim and the University of Illinois asked volunteers to hold a pen either in their teeth, like a dog with a bone, which required activating some of the same muscles involved in smiling; or in their lips, as if they were sucking on a straw, which activated frowning muscles. Then they were asked to rate how funny a series of *Far Side* cartoons were. Sure enough, the subjects rated the cartoons as funnier, by about one point on a 10-point scale, when they were (sort of) smiling. This illustrates what's known as the "facial feedback" hypothesis, an idea that can be traced back to Charles Darwin: just as emotions trigger a physical response, that physical response can amplify or perhaps even create the corresponding emotion. Related experiments have extended this finding to clusters of related mental states: smiling, for instance, makes you happier, but it also enhances feelings of safety and—intriguingly—cognitive ease, a concept intimately tied to effort.

Does that also apply to the effort of exercise? Marcora used EMG electrodes to record the activity of facial muscles while subjects lifted leg weights or cycled, and found a strong link between reported effort and the activation of frowning muscles during heavy exercise. A subsequent study by Taiwanese researchers also linked jaw-clenching muscles to effort. It's no coincidence, then, that coaches have long instructed runners to "relax your face" or "relax your jaw." One of the most famous proponents of facial relaxation was the legendary sprint coach Bud Winter, who had honed his ideas while training pilots during World War II. "Watch his lower lip," Winter instructed a *Sports Illustrated* reporter who visited one of his practices in 1959, as his star sprinter streaked past. "If his lower lip is relaxed and flopping when he runs, his upper body is loose." Then Winter offered a firsthand demonstration of the optimal running face. "Like that," he said, flicking his tension-free lower lip with his fingers. "It's got to be loose."

In fact, smiles and other facial expressions can have even more subtle effects, as one of Marcora's most remarkable experiments showed. With his colleagues Anthony Blanchfield and James Hardy, of Bangor University in Wales, he paid thirteen volunteers to pedal a stationary bike at a predetermined pace for as long as they could. Such time-to-exhaustion trials are a well-established method of measuring physical limits, but in this case there was also a hidden psychological component. As the cyclists pedaled, a screen in front of them periodically flashed images of happy or sad faces in imperceptible 16-millisecond bursts, ten to twenty times shorter than a typical blink. The cyclists who were shown sad faces rode, on average, for just over 22 minutes. Those who were shown happy faces rode for three minutes longer and reported a lower sense of effort at corresponding time points. Seeing a smiling face, even subliminally, evokes feelings of ease that bleed into your perception of how hard you're working at other tasks, like pedaling a bike.

With these results in mind, the idea that sports psychology can also alter your sense of effort no longer seems quite so far-fetched. To prove it, Marcora and his colleagues tested a simple self-talk intervention—precisely the approach my teammates and I had laughed at two decades earlier. They had twenty-four volunteers complete a cycling test to exhaustion, then gave half of them some simple guidance on how to use positive self-talk before another cycling test two weeks later. The self-talk group learned to use certain phrases early on ("feeling good!") and others later in a race or workout ("push through this!"), and practiced using the phrases during training to figure out which ones felt most comfortable and effective. Sure enough, in the second cycling test, the self-talk group lasted 18 percent longer than the control group, and their rating of perceived exertion climbed more slowly throughout the test. Just like a smile or frown, the words in your head have the power to influence the very feelings they're supposed to reflect.

As Marcora and his fellow motorcyclists rumbled across Europe and Central Asia, they were gradually becoming fitter: losing weight, increasing grip strength, gaining aerobic fitness. But they were also getting increasingly tired. Before and after each day's ride, Marcora administered a Psychomotor Vigilance Test to his subjects, who had to tap a button as quickly as possible on a small handheld device in response to an irregular series of flashing lights. On average, their reaction time slowed from about 300 milliseconds in the morning to 350 milliseconds after nine or more hours in the saddle—a significant decrease if you're whipping around a blind corner on a mountain road or swerving to avoid a wandering goat. The decline was most pronounced as they crossed the Tibetan plateau, where the thin air magnified the effects of mental fatigue: average end-of-ride scores on the Psychomotor Vigilance Test ballooned to 450 milliseconds.

Fortunately, Marcora had a potent countermeasure. Tucked into his pannier of lab equipment was a stash of Military Energy Gum, a chewing gum containing 100 milligrams of caffeine that is quickly absorbed through the inner lining of your mouth. Half of the gums were the standard-issue rocket fuel; the other half were specially prepared caffeine-free placebos. Starting after lunch each day, Marcora chewed six pieces of gum, having organized and disguised them so that even he didn't know if he was getting caffeine or not that day. When he crunched the data after the trip, the results were striking: the slowdown in reaction time between the beginning and end of the day was completely eliminated on the days his gum contained caffeine.

Caffeine's perk-up powers aren't exactly a secret—without even considering coffee, caffeine pills are already one of the most widely used legal supplements among athletes—but the results illustrate how, in Marcora's view, everything comes down to the perception of effort. There are several theories about how caffeine boosts strength and endurance. Some argue it directly enhances muscle contraction; others suggest it enhances fat oxidation to provide extra metabolic energy. To Marcora, the most convincing explanation relates to caffeine's ability to shut down receptors in the brain that detect the presence of adenosine, a "neuromodulator" molecule associated with mental fatigue. Warding off mental fatigue, in turn, keeps your sense of effort lower, allowing you to exert yourself harder and longer.

The demands of riding a motorcycle may seem far removed from typical tests of endurance, but in fact they closely mimic the demands encountered by soldiers, Marcora points out. In both cases, you have to maintain high levels of focus and concentration for hours at a time while doing moderate physical activity in bulky, poorly ventilated gear. And in both cases, even a brief lapse can be fatal. As a result, much of the funding for Marcora's research, from caffeine gum to "brain endurance training," comes from Britain's Ministry of Defence, who are interested in ways of fighting both mental and physical fatigue.

Closely linked to the sustained attention required by adventure motorcyclists and soldiers is another cognitive process called "response inhibition"—the ability to consciously override your impulses. This is one of the skills that Stanford University psychologist Walter Mischel tested with his famous "marshmallow test" in the late 1960s. The experimenters offered preschoolers a choice between one treat right away, or two treats if they waited for fifteen minutes. Over decades of follow-up, the children who resisted temptation the longest ended up with better test scores, more education, and lower body-mass index. Other studies have linked low response inhibition to higher risk of outcomes like divorce and even crack cocaine addiction.

No one has checked whether the kids who aced the marshmallow test were more likely to become champion endurance athletes—but they should. For motorcyclists and soldiers, impulse inhibition matters because you have to suppress the urge to let your mind wander, and a similar challenge faces marathoners and other endurance athletes. Think of it this way: If you stick your finger in a candle flame, your natural response will be to yank it out as soon as you start feeling heat. The essence of pushing to your limits in endurance sports is learning to override that instinct so that you can hold your finger a little closer to the flame—and keep it there, not for seconds but for minutes or even hours.

Marcora and his colleagues tested this idea in an experiment in 2014, using a technique called the Stroop task to tax their subjects' response inhibition. The task involves words flashing on a screen in various colors; you have to press a particular button in response to each color. What's tricky is that the words themselves are colors: you might see the word *green* in blue letters, and you have to overcome your initial impulse to press the button corresponding to green instead of blue. In the study, subjects performed the task twice: once with the words and colors mismatched, requiring response inhibition, and once with the words and colors matched, as a control. In both cases, after 30 minutes of the cognitive task, they ran a 5K as fast as possible on a treadmill.

The results were clear. Even though the subjects weren't aware of any mental fatigue, they started their 5K slower after the response inhibition version of the task, rated their level of effort higher throughout the run, and finished with times 6 percent slower. That suggests that response inhibition really is an important mental component of endurance—and that it's a finite resource that runs low if you use it too much. Holding your finger to the flame (or simply focusing on a tricky computer task) takes mental effort, and that effort is just as real as the effort of moving your legs.

It has long been a cliché that the best athletes are defined as much by their superior minds as by their muscle. With response inhibition, we have a way of testing this, which is what a team based at the University of Canberra and the neighboring Australian Institute of Sport, working with Marcora, decided to do. They recruited eleven elite professional cyclists and compared them with nine trained amateur cyclists. All the volunteers completed two 20-minute time trials, one preceded by a 30-minute Stroop task to deplete their response inhibition, the other preceded by a control task of simply gazing at a black cross on a white screen for 10 minutes.

The first interesting finding was that the professionals were significantly better at the Stroop task, amassing an average of 705 correct responses during the 30-minute test compared to 576 for the amateurs. In other words, to the list of measurable traits that distinguish the pros from the rest of us—the size of their heart, the number of capillaries feeding their muscles, their lactate threshold, and so on—we can now add response inhibition.

The second interesting finding was how the cyclists performed in the time trial after completing the response-inhibiting Stroop task. The amateurs, depleted by the mental effort of focusing on all those flashing letters, produced 4.4 percent less power than in their control ride. The pros, on the other hand, didn't slow down at all. They were able to resist the effects of mental fatigue, at least in the doses produced by a 30-minute Stroop task, and cycle just as fast as when they were fresh.

There are two ways to explain these findings. One is that the pros were born with superior response inhibition and resistance to mental fatigue, and that's one of the reasons they've ended up as elite athletes. The other is that long years of training help the mind adapt to resist mental fatigue, just as the body adapts to resist physical fatigue. Which is it? I suspect a bit of both, and the smattering of evidence that exists supports the idea that these traits are partly inherited but also can be improved with training. And this, in turn, raises the really big question: What's the best way to boost your mental endurance? Marcora's idea, as he proposed back in 2011 at the conference in Bathurst, is that specially tailored cognitive challenges like the Stroop task, repeated over and over, constitute a form of "brain endurance training" that can give athletes an edge. As I'll describe in Chapter 11, I visited the University of Kent for a brain-training boot camp, and then tried out the technique for twelve weeks while preparing for a marathon. Marcora has also run a series of military-funded trials of the technique—and the initial results suggest he's onto something big.

The studies described in this chapter make it clear that we can't talk about the limits of endurance without considering the brain and perception of effort. But they don't necessarily mean that Marcora's psychobiological theory is right. In fact, not everyone agrees his theory is even new. Tim Noakes, when I asked him about Marcora's ideas in 2010, dismissed them as a minor variation of his own central governor model: "The only distinction between our model and his model—and he has to differentiate, obviously—is that everything is consciously controlled," he said.

The distinction between conscious and unconscious has become a bitterly contested flashpoint between the two camps, but the differences aren't as great as they appear. Marcora does indeed argue that the decision to speed up, slow down, or stop is always conscious and voluntary. But such "decisions," he acknowledges, can be effectively forced on you by an intolerably high sense of effort. And crucially, they can still be influenced by any number of factors that you're not consciously aware of, as demonstrated most clearly by his own experiment with subliminal images. Noakes and his colleagues, on the other side, don't dispute the importance of effort, motivation, and conscious decision making. When you run a marathon, it's not the central governor that prevents you from sprinting for the first 100 meters (a fact demonstrated by the enthusiastic souls who do, in fact, sprint at the start of marathons and later pay the price).

It's true, though, that there are some real contrasts between Noakes's and Marcora's theories, and they're most obvious at the limits of total exhaustion—a state most people rarely, if ever, encounter. Imagine going to the gym, setting the treadmill to 10 miles per hour, and deciding to run for as long as you can. For most people, the decision to step off will be purely voluntary, a simple result of the effort becoming greater than they're willing to tolerate. But if, instead, you're running the final mile of the Olympic marathon, neck-and-neck with a rival for the gold medal, it's harder to accept that the runner who slackens first does so because the effort feels too great or because she's not motivated enough. Noakes would argue that the runner's brain is overriding her conscious desires, reducing muscle recruitment in order to prevent damage to critical organs—and that process is not only unconscious, but is flatly contradicting the runner's conscious decisions. To anyone who has raced seriously, it's the latter explanation that *feels* right.

Of course, the other option is that such scenarios of truly maximal effort and motivation push you to plain old physical limits—that, as A. V. Hill would have argued nearly a century ago, it's muscle fatigue or the limits of oxygen delivery that hold you back in the final mile of the Olympics. When I first started planning this book, in 2009, it was going to be all about Tim Noakes and how his ideas had upended the conventional body-centric view of endurance. Then I discovered Marcora's work, and realized that no explanation of endurance could be complete without considering the psychology involved. And then, as I dug deeper, I got to know some of the physiologists who don't believe either of them, and whose views of human endurance are still rooted in the heart, lungs, and muscles—like University of Exeter physiologist Andrew Jones, who helped guide Paula Radcliffe to a marathon world record and whose Breaking2 lab data suggests Eliud Kipchoge is capable of a sub-two-hour run. And I discovered that they, too, have some powerful evidence to back their views.

So who is right? The short answer is that scientists are currently fighting about it, strenuously and sometimes bitterly, with no end in sight. The longer—and to me, more interesting—answer is that, as the comparison above between running on a treadmill in the gym and racing in the Olympics illustrates, it depends. In Part II of the book, we'll explore how specific factors like pain, oxygen, heat, thirst, and fuel define your limits in different contexts. We'll encounter situations that seem to confirm Noakes's view, like sports drinks that boost your endurance even if you don't swallow them. We'll explore whether it's really possible for a panicked mother to lift a car off her child. And we'll see what happens when an injection in the spine temporarily removes the limits imposed by the brain, allowing athletes to push their muscles all the way to the brink—a dream scenario that turns out to be more of a nightmare.

Two Hours

November 30, 2016

A homeless man is asleep in the doorway, his grungy brown sleeping bag zipped up to his nose to keep the drizzle off. Next to his head, stowed neatly out of the weather, is a crisp, spotless pair of brightly colored Nike trainers with fluorescent yellow laces. This, I tell myself, is peak Portland. I jog a few more blocks back to my downtown hotel, shower up, and head out with David Willey to the manicured mega-campus of Nike World Headquarters to find out how, exactly, the company plans to leapfrog a half-century ahead of my predicted marathon timeline.

It's immediately clear that the Breaking2 project isn't just a passing whim cooked up by the marketing department. As we're ushered through security into the Nike Sport Research Lab—an area, our escorts breathlessly assure us, that is strictly off-limits even to the vast majority of Nike employees on the site—we pass a massive mural at the end of a hallway that doubles as a two-lane rubberized running track. It reads, in pixelated scoreboard font, "1:59:59." Some twenty people have been working on the secret project, more or less full-time, for nearly two years, with a total cost that the company won't disclose but clearly extends to millions, if not tens of millions, of dollars.

The barrier-breaking science behind the plan? You name it, they're willing to try it. In a series of meetings that stretches late into the evening, we hear from the company's top physiologists, biomechanists, and product designers about the lengths they've gone to in contemplating how to squeeze extra inches from exhausted muscles. Some of the crazier ideas have, perhaps mercifully, been left on the cutting-room floor—like pinning your arms to your sides to save wasted motion and energy. Tests on former elite runner Matt Tegenkamp using a specially designed elastic sling showed a measurable efficiency boost, but "he wouldn't wear it," Matthew Nurse, the lab's director, tells us. "It looked like a *Three Stooges* episode." The footwear team, meanwhile, had contemplated a stripped-down "track spike for the marathon," including one prototype with the heel completely eliminated to save weight. There was just one problem: the runners who tried it hated it.

In the end, the team zeroed in on five key areas: selecting the best athletes, optimizing the course and environment, executing the best possible training, delivering the right fuel and hydration, and deploying cutting-edge shoes and apparel. For each of these pillars, they take us through how they think they can improve on Dennis Kimetto's 2:02:57. In some cases, the gains are admittedly marginal. Switching from loose shorts to half-tights, adding textured dimples to the singlet, and sticking aerodynamic tape to the calves—altogether an overhaul of the marathoner's typical clothing might save "between one and 60 seconds" over the course of a marathon, apparel physiologist Dan Judelson tells me. "But even if it's just one second, that would be significant. We would feel really bad if we didn't try everything and they ran 2:00:01."

The big gains, from what I am gathering, will come from two sources. First, they have a new shoe with a counterintuitively thick, cushioned sole made with an advanced foam that breaks all previous records for lightness and resilience. Embedded in the sole is a curved carbon-fiber plate that adds enough stiffness to avoid the energy loss that would otherwise result from running in such a marshmallowy shoe. External tests secretly conducted at the University of Colorado show that the shoe improves efficiency by about 4 percent on average—a stunning figure that will spark fierce controversy when the shoe is unveiled publicly. People either don't believe such a big gain is possible, or, if they do, they think it should be banned. But for now, the shoes don't break any existing rules—and I begin, for the first time, to seriously contemplate the possibility that Nike's mission might have a chance of succeeding.

The second big factor is drafting. In my 2014 analysis, I had argued that the cost of overcoming air resistance, even on a perfectly still day, might amount to 100 seconds over the course of a two-hour marathon. That might seem far-fetched—until you remember that the runners will be sustaining a pace of about 4:35 per mile, which for most of us is essentially a sprint. Studies dating back to the 1970s have suggested that running directly behind another runner can eliminate most of this extra effort, but in practice it's difficult to draft that closely behind someone else. And to pace a two-hour marathon all the way to the finish, you'd need someone—or preferably several people—who can run a two-hour marathon themselves, since world-record rules forbid having fresh pacers jump in partway through the race. Nike's solution: give up on the idea of setting an official world record, so that they can deploy a large team of pacemakers who will rotate in and out of the race in order to pace the chosen ones all the way to the finish.

None of this matters, of course, if the athletes running the race aren't already in near-world-record shape. The Breaking2 team, along with expert outside consultants like Andrew Jones, has spent eighteen months bringing some of the best athletes in the world to the lab for comprehensive testing, including the three key parameters—VO_2max, running economy, and lactate threshold—that Michael Joyner highlighted in 1991.

Jones, a dapper and soft-spoken Welshman, is perhaps best known for his work with marathon great Paula Radcliffe, whom he began advising when she was a precocious teenager and he was a graduate student. In 2002, when Radcliffe was preparing for her marathon debut, he told her she was ready to run 2:18—a bold view given that the world record was 2:18:47. She went on to run 2:18:56 in London. Later that year, before the Chicago Marathon, he predicted a 2:17; she ran 2:17:18. Finally, the next spring, her lab values indicated a 2:16—and she ran 2:15:25 in London, which is still the world record. A. V. Hill would have been proud.

Jones's experiences with Radcliffe give him—and me, as I listen to his briefing in Beaverton—confidence in the power of treadmill testing to predict seemingly improbable results. But they also underscore other necessary intangibles. "Her capacity to hurt herself was unprecedented," he says. So in addition to treadmill testing, test runs on the track, and detailed analysis of athletes' racing history, the Breaking2 team also made more gut-level assessments. They considered the athletes' swagger, their response to challenges, and other elements of attitude and outlook that might make or break the mission.

The three men they've selected, who are all here in Beaverton for further testing and to launch their training for the race, are a mix of obvious and surprising choices. At thirty-two, Eliud Kipchoge is the reigning Olympic champion, the third-fastest marathoner in history, and the consensus best marathoner on the planet at the moment. Zersenay Tadese, a thirty-four-year-old Eritrean runner, is the world-record holder for the half-marathon, and according to an earlier study is among the most efficient runners ever tested in a lab. Lelisa Desisa, a twenty-six-year-old Ethiopian, is a two-time Boston Marathon champion who has proven to be a gritty competitor in head-to-head races.

Over the next few days, we watch as the scientific team puts the runners through their paces. One by one, they run in a cold chamber set to 50 degrees in shorts and singlet, with eight wireless thermometers taped to various parts of their body to assess their response to the cool conditions they hope for on race day. They try different versions of the prototype shoe, while the scientists measure their efficiency, to personalize the stiffness of the carbon-fiber plate for each runner. When Kipchoge tiptoes with exaggerated care onto the treadmill, one of the scientists edges around to the back of the machine, ready to be a spotter if needed. It's only the second time Kipchoge has run on a treadmill—the first time was during the initial selection process—and it's hard not to think of Bambi flailing around on the ice. Kipchoge's lab data, Jones later confides, was surprisingly ordinary, presumably because he was so uncomfortable on the treadmill. For the Olympic champion, they decided to look past this mediocre lab data.

Thanks to the language barrier, it's hard to get a read on what Tadese and Desisa think of all this. Through interpreters, they gamely field our questions, but all that we really come away with is the sense that they think running a two-hour marathon will be really hard, but with help (and presumably big piles of money) from Nike, they're willing to give it a shot. Kipchoge, whose English is fluent, is different. Though he's so soft-spoken that you have to lean forward and squint to hear him, his words—and his demeanor, and the aura that David and I later agree he exudes—reveal a serene and imperturbable confidence. Is this what winning an Olympic gold medal does for you, I wonder? Or is it what you need to get there in the first place?

After a week in Portland, the athletes disperse back to their homes in Kenya, Eritrea, and Ethiopia. All three men, like the vast majority of the world's best distance runners these days, were born, grew up, and train in the East African highlands along the Great Rift Valley, at elevations of at least 6,000 feet above sea level. The thin, oxygen-poor air at these heights makes running harder and triggers adaptations like an increase in the number of red blood cells available to shuttle oxygen from the lungs to working muscles. In fact, anyone born into this environment carries oxygen-sparing traits like enhanced lung volume with them for the rest of their lives. Shalane Flanagan, the second-fastest women's marathoner in U.S. history, was born in Boulder (elevation 5,430 feet); Ryan Hall, the fastest American-born men's marathoner, grew up in Big Bear Lake (elevation 6,752).

In late January, a twelve-person team from Nike embarks on a two-week trip to visit Kipchoge, Desisa, and Tadese in their home training environments. The contrast between the high-tech pursuit of marginal gains and the simple life and elemental grind of African marathon training is striking. "It's very humbling to see the Olympic champion hauling up cold water in a bucket from a well after his workout," Philip Skiba, one of the outside scientific consultants working with the Breaking2 team, tells me when I check in by phone during the Kenyan leg.

The purpose of the trip is partly to build trust with the athletes, but there's also science on the agenda. Lead physiologist Brett Kirby and his team have rigged up a makeshift wearable wind-speed meter to help the athletes get a sense of exactly where they need to run to get the most benefit from drafting behind other runners. They have a portable ultrasound device that estimates how much carbohydrate is stored in leg muscles, which they deploy before and after long runs to assess how quickly these reserves are being depleted. And they also have muscle oxygenation sensors that the athletes wear during hard workouts at two-hour marathon pace; this data, Jones tells me, suggests that Kipchoge—like Clarence DeMar at the Harvard Fatigue Lab almost a century ago—is in a sustainable state of "stable physiology" at this pace.

One of the most urgent items on the agenda is figuring out exactly what and how much the athletes should drink during the race. Instead of aid tables every five kilometers, as is standard in big-city marathons, the Breaking2 team plans to ride alongside the athletes on a bike—saving, they estimate, about seven seconds per bottle handoff—and distribute drinks every three kilometers or so. The goal is to keep the athletes fueled by providing 60 to 90 grams of carbohydrate per hour, which is far more than the athletes are used to. This is no easy task, given that it's the carbohydrate equivalent of scarfing down about four cups of cooked spaghetti during the race, so it takes practice. During one 22-mile run, the scientists drive behind Desisa and offer him drinks periodically. In a debriefing the next day, Desisa reports feeling that he had drunk "a lot" during the run—but in fact, he had consumed just 400 of the 1,500 milliliters of sports drink he'd been given.

By the end of the trip, the team is feeling cautiously optimistic as they chip away at the various physiological barriers—muscle, oxygen, heat, thirst, fuel—that stand between the runners and a two-hour marathon. Meanwhile, from Kipchoge's perspective, there's a more subtle transformation under way. When I reach him by phone at his training camp near the town of Kaptagat, I ask him what he's doing differently to prepare for the epic task ahead. His most recent race, after all, was a 59:44 half-marathon win in Delhi; soon he'll have to double the distance at nearly the same pace. The physical training won't change from previous years, he tells me—"but my mind will be different." To him, the challenge is primarily mental, and the widespread skepticism that has greeted the attempt is, in some ways, a failure of imagination. "Most of the people were saying they will die before they see a man running under two hours," he admits when I ask what other runners in Kenya think. "But I think I will prove them wrong."

To do so, though, won't simply be a matter of surmounting physiological limits and displaying psychological strength. Kipchoge, inevitably and excruciatingly, will have to suffer.

Part II

LIMITS

CHAPTER 5

Pain

From the very start of the very first stage of the 2014 Tour de France, which that year traversed the rugged moors of Yorkshire, Jens Voigt was on the attack. At forty-two, the German veteran was the oldest rider in the race, competing in his record-tying seventeenth straight Tour. But his presence, he seemed to be saying, was not merely ornamental. He and two other riders quickly broke away from the peloton, opening up a gap as they charged toward the first climb of the day. With more than 100 miles to go before the finish, it was highly unlikely that the trio would manage to stay ahead of the peloton—but such brazen, long-odds attacks were exactly what had turned a modest journeyman like Voigt into a cult figure among cycling fans.

At the top of the first climb, however, reality intruded. His two breakaway companions easily gapped him by a few bike lengths to claim the points for best climber, and he realized that he wouldn't be able to outsprint them in subsequent climbs or at the finish. His team director, over the radio, suggested that he drop back to conserve energy. "I said, 'No, no, no, the other way around! If I want the mountain jersey, I have to go now,'" Voigt recalled after the race. So he redoubled his efforts, dropped the other two riders before the next climb, and—while he was eventually caught by the peloton—ended up claiming the polka-dot jersey for best climber as well as the stage's most combative rider award. All in all, it was a vintage performance for the man whose trademarked catchphrase, coined when a Danish television reporter asked how he handled the fatigue of his characteristic breakaways, is "Shut up, legs!"

While great riders are often distinguished by the extremes of their physiology or their grace in the saddle, Voigt's singular characteristic during an eighteen-year professional career was his appetite for suffering. His "open acknowledgment of pain as a state of mind to be combated, repressed and ultimately overcome," *Cycling Weekly* opined, "is perhaps part of the reason he is revered by cycling fans as the hardman of the peloton." Voigt himself believed that his struggles to make the cut in the rigorous elite sports academies of his East German youth left a long-lasting mark: "I think that over all these years, I learned to set my pain threshold higher than other people's," he reflected in his autobiography (title: *Shut Up, Legs!*). "I think I have a pain threshold that is 10 to 20 percent higher than most others. I don't know if you can scientifically prove it, but I totally believe it."

In the popular imagination (and the thesaurus), endurance and suffering are inextricably linked. "No pain, no gain" is a motto across most sports, but in skill sports this relationship is more negotiable, says Wolfgang Freund, a researcher at University Hospitals Ulm in Germany who studies pain in athletes. The incomparable Argentine soccer star Diego Maradona, for example, "at least had the illusion that a brilliant soccer player didn't need to suffer," he says. For cyclists and other endurance athletes, though, pain is unavoidable, and how you handle it is intimately tied to how well you perform. In 2013, Freund published a telling study on the pain tolerance of ultra-endurance runners competing in the TransEurope Footrace, an epic pain-fest in which participants covered 2,789 miles over 64 days with no rest days. He asked eleven of the competitors to dunk their hands in ice water for three minutes; by the end, they rated the pain as about 6 out of 10 on average. In contrast, the nonathlete control group gave up after an average of just 96 seconds when their pain maxed out at 10; only three of them even completed the test.

Such findings reinforce the idea that, all else being equal, the gold medal goes to whoever is willing to suffer a bit more than everyone else. Freund isn't the only one to find that well-trained athletes can tolerate more pain; others have shown that regular physical training, especially if it involves unpleasant high-intensity workouts, increases your pain tolerance. But the link between what's happening in your muscles and what you feel in your head turns out to be much more indirect than you might assume. "Pain is more than one thing," says Dr. Jeffrey Mogil, the head of the Pain Genetics Lab at McGill University. It's a sensation, like vision or touch; it's an emotion, like anger or sadness; and it's also a "drive state" that compels action, like hunger. For athletes, the role of pain depends on how these different effects mingle together in their specific situation. Sometimes pain slows them to a halt; other times it drives them to even greater heights.

Much of Voigt's career was spent suffering for the greater glory of his team leaders—Jan Ullrich at the 2000 Olympic; Ivan Basso, Andy Schleck, and others at the Grand Tours. Cycling is a sport with intricate team tactics, where the crucial impact of aerodynamics and topography mean that place is everything and times have little meaning. But there is one major exception—one challenge that strips away these extraneous details and simply asks: How far can you pedal your bicycle in sixty minutes? And how much are you willing to hurt to do it? So, as he contemplated his final season as a professional in 2014, it was fitting, if not inevitable, that Voigt would choose to make his last race an assault on the Hour, as the sixty-minutes-of-cycling record is reverentially referred to. "The beauty of it lies in its simplicity," he explained. "It's one bike, one rider, one gear. There are no tactics, no teammates, no bonus seconds at the finish. The hour record is just about how much pain you can handle! It's the hour of truth."

The first official Hour record, at 35.325 kilometers (just under 22 miles), was set in 1893 at Paris's storied Vélodrome Buffalo track (so named because Buffalo Bill's circus had performed on the site). The inaugural record holder was the domineering journalist and impresario Henri Desgrange, who a decade later founded the Tour de France. In the years that followed, attempts on the Hour became a rite of passage for would-be legends of the sport, and a source of endless stories:

the two Frenchmen who batted the record back and forth five times in three years before World War I, always careful not to break it by so much that future record attempts (and the attendant payouts) would be out of reach; Italian star Fausto Coppi's unlikely 1942 ride in Milan, amid the chaos and bombing of World War II; Jacques Anquetil's unofficial record in 1967, unratified because he was asked to provide a post-race urine sample for drug testing—a new innovation at the time—and indignantly declined.

The most iconic record of all came in 1972, capping the finest year of racing by the man most fans acknowledge as the greatest cyclist of them all, the Belgian Eddie Merckx. Merckx's Hour attempt, held in the thin air of Mexico City in late October, was his 139th race of the year. He'd won 51 of them, including the overall titles at the Tour de France and the Giro d'Italia; it was only thanks to a saddle sore picked up during the Tour that he had backed off his rigorous racing schedule enough to make some brief preparations for his assault on the record.

Merckx decided that if he was going to take the trouble of flying all the way to a mountaintop velodrome with a specially built track bike, he might as well knock off the world records at shorter distances on the way. "Excellent," he replied when friends warned how unreasonably fast he would have to start. "I must suffer during the opening kilometers." And so it was that, after a few rain-soaked days of delay, Merckx set off so quickly that his times at 1K and 5K were world-class, and he set new world records at 10K and 20K—and he wasn't even halfway through. Inevitably, the laps slowed as Merckx's anguish mounted, and he began to squirm in the saddle. He finished, in the end, with 49,431 meters (just under 31 miles), almost half a mile clear of the previous mark, held by Danish rider Ole Ritter. When he dismounted from his bike, as cycling journalist Michael Hutchinson recounts, he was a wreck: "He couldn't move. He couldn't speak. When finally he strung a few words together, it was to say that it had been terrible. No one who had not done it could know what it was like."

Watching archival footage of Merckx's performance, it's clear that his pain was viscerally real. But did he really suffer more than Ritter—

or than Lagrange eighty years earlier; or than British journalist and cycling fan Simon Usborne when he managed 42,879 meters while writing a feature about the Hour in 2015 (the agony, like "death without dying," left him feeling for days like he had aged by thirty years, he reported); or than any man or woman off the street would if he or she decided to pedal as hard as possible for an hour? Like many bits of folk wisdom, there is at least a kernel of truth here.

Among the first to study pain perception in athletes was Karel Gijsbers, a psychologist at the University of Stirling, in Scotland, who (with a graduate student) published an influential paper in the *British Journal of Medicine* in 1981. He put 30 elite swimmers from the Scottish national team through a series of pain tests, and compared their results to 30 club-level swimmers and 26 nonathletes. The protocol involved cutting off circulation to the subjects' arms with a blood-pressure cuff, then having them clench and unclench their fist once per second. "Pain threshold" was defined as the number of contractions needed to produce a sensation that registered as pain rather than merely discomfort; "pain tolerance" was quantified as the total number of contractions before the subject gave up.

The first finding was that pain threshold was essentially the same in all three groups, starting after around 50 contractions. As Merckx would undoubtedly attest, top athletes are not immune to pain; they feel it like everyone else. But there were dramatic differences in pain *tolerance:* the national-team swimmers endured an average of 132 contractions before calling for mercy, compared to 89 in the club swimmers and 70 in the nonathletes. The differences, Gijsbers suggested, must result from the systematic exposure to intense but intermittent pain during training—perhaps by harnessing brain chemicals like endorphins, or perhaps simply thanks to psychological coping mechanisms. "It is reported," he noted drily, "that pain can be strangely satisfying to the highly motivated athlete."

Subsequent studies have mostly confirmed these findings: athletes, and especially endurance athletes, are consistently willing to tolerate more pain. Like Wolfgang Freund's study of TransEurope runners, the results pose a chicken-and-egg question: do great athletes learn to endure more pain, or is their greatness a consequence of naturally high pain tolerance? While the truth undoubtedly lies somewhere between those two options, a curious footnote in Gijsbers's results points toward the former. He retested the elite swimmers at three different times of year and found that they scored highest on the pain tolerance test in June, during their peak racing season; lowest in October, after their off-season; and somewhere in the middle during their regular training period in March.

These seasonal fluctuations suggest that pain tolerance is linked to the type of training you're doing—and that's exactly what researchers Martyn Morris and Thomas O'Leary, of Oxford Brookes University in Britain, confirmed in a 2017 study. They used the same pain protocol as Gijsbers—fist-clenching with no circulation to the arm—before, during, and after a six-week training period during which volunteers did either medium-intensity continuous cycling or high-intensity interval workouts. The training programs were matched to require roughly the same amount of work, and both groups increased their fitness, as measured by VO_2max and lactate threshold, by the same amount.

But there were two key differences between the groups. First, pain tolerance increased by 41 percent in the high-intensity group, while the medium-intensity subjects didn't see any change. This shows that simply getting fitter doesn't magically increase your pain tolerance; *how* you get fit matters: you have to suffer. Second, despite the similar fitness gains, the high-intensity group saw much bigger improvements in their racing performance, as measured by a series of time-to-exhaustion tests at different intensities. In one test, the interval group lasted 148 percent longer on the bike, compared to a mere 38 percent gain for the medium-intensity trainers. Intriguingly, the individual improvements in the time-to-exhaustion tests were correlated with the individual gains in pain tolerance, meaning that the cyclists who learned to handle more pain from the tourniquet test were the same ones who managed to cycle faster.

This is a profound finding: pain in training leads to greater tourniquet tolerance, and greater tourniquet tolerance predicts better race performance. Many athletes, of course, make this link intuitively. Triathlete Jesse Thomas, for example, learned to use his deep-tissue massage sessions as a form of pain training: "When I'm hurting like crazy," he explains, "instead of blocking out the pain, I try to accept it, feel it as much as possible." Morris and O'Leary's study will need to be replicated by other groups under different conditions before its results can be fully confirmed. But it suggests that, at least in recreational athletes, pain tolerance is both a trainable trait and a limiting factor in endurance. And it leaves a ripe and juicy question dangling for future researchers: can you get faster by simply training yourself to better tolerate or block out pain?

The beauty of the Hour record stems, in part, from its simplicity. But even the simplest idea can be enveloped in smothering layers of bureaucratic regulations and seemingly arbitrary diktats. After aerodynamic advances in bike construction and rider position helped the record advance by 10 percent, to 56 kilometers, over a three-year period in the 1990s, the International Cycling Union (known by its French acronym, UCI) decided to crack down. In 2000, they wiped the record books clean and restored Eddie Merckx as record holder, declaring that all future attempts would have to be made with Merckx-vintage bikes with wire spokes and round-tubed frames.

One of the more curious new stipulations was that only one person would be allowed on the track to give feedback to the rider attempting the record. Another prohibited modern timekeeping aids, wristwatches included. These two surprises, unwritten in any set of official rules, were sprung by a UCI official on an unsuspecting Michael Hutchinson, the cycling journalist and champion time trialist, moments before the start of his own attempt on the Hour in 2003. He was also not permitted to wear his heart-rate monitor, and even the digital lap counter alongside the track was disabled—a handicap that

Hutchinson only discovered after the attempt had started, meaning that he had no means of gauging how far or long he'd cycled, or how his body was responding. Hamstrung by these unexpected restrictions, he abandoned the attempt after 40 minutes.

These and other rules killed interest in the record for over a decade, until the UCI loosened the rules again in 2014. The fortunate timing is what made it possible for the forty-three-year-old Voigt to attempt the record as his retirement ride, despite being years past his prime. He could use a modern time-trial bike to chase a retro record that was, by 2014, still only a few hundred meters longer than Merckx's 1972 ride. But most of the restrictive rules on external feedback—one person on the track, no power meters, no heart-rate monitors, and so on—remained in effect. Even glancing up at a stadium scoreboard would require breaking out of the aerodynamic riding position. The perfect ride, then, would be like floating in a sensory deprivation tank for 60 minutes. To gauge his effort and ride at the outer edge of his limits, Voigt would have to embrace the pain, feel it, and read it like a carefully calibrated speedometer.

The idea that pain might actually be *helpful* is not particularly intuitive. What cyclist or rower or runner hasn't, at some point, wished for immunity from mid-race pain? And it's certainly true that, in some cases at least, blocking pain can boost endurance. In 2010, a team of researchers led by Alexis Mauger, who was then at the University of Exeter, in Britain, showed that giving well-trained cyclists 1,500 milligrams of acetaminophen—plain old Tylenol—boosted their performance in a 10-mile time trial by about 2 percent compared to when they were given a placebo. The drugged cyclists were able to push to a higher heart rate and accumulate higher levels of lactate in their blood, while their perceived effort remained the same as during the placebo ride. Less pain made the effort feel easier, allowing the cyclists to push closer to their true physiological limits, the researchers argued.

This is one of those "new" insights from the lab that has been conventional wisdom in the peloton more or less since the penny-farthing era. Early holders of the Hour record were unabashed about the need for pharmaceutical aid. When Fausto Coppi, who set the record in 1942, was asked if he took drugs during his career, he said, "Yes, whenever it was necessary." And when was it necessary? "Almost always." Coppi, like Jacques Anquetil a generation later, relied mostly on amphetamines, which provide an in-the-moment boost. But painkillers, too, had a role. Frenchman Roger Rivière set Hour records in 1957 and 1958; but just two years later, while racing down a steep descent during the Tour de France, he lost control and flipped over a low wall, falling sixty feet into a ravine and breaking two vertebrae, leaving him paralyzed for the rest of his short life (he died of cancer at forty). Doctors reportedly found painkillers in his pockets and in his bloodstream. He initially claimed his brakes had failed, but later admitted he had taken Palfium, an opioid reported to be three times more potent than morphine, to dull the pain. He was so numb, a friend reported, that he had been unable to pull his brake levers.

There are other reasons to avoid dulling the pain too much. In a series of experiments starting in 2009, researcher Markus Amann, then at the University of Wisconsin, investigated what happens to cyclists when they can't feel pain at all. Amann and his colleagues injected the nerve blocker fentanyl into the spines of their volunteers, preventing signals from traveling up from the leg muscles to the brain, and asked them to ride 5K as hard as they could on a stationary bike. The effects were dramatic. The volunteers had been given a gift that many athletes dream of—the ability to push as hard as they wanted without feeling pain—and they took advantage of the opportunity to ride themselves into a smoking ruin. By the end of the time trial, the riders couldn't even get off the bikes by themselves. Some couldn't even unclip their feet from the pedals, Amann recalls, "and not a single one was able to walk."

But the results told a different, and unexpected, story. Despite their temporary superhuman status, the subjects didn't ride any faster than when they received a placebo injection, thanks to erratic and overly ambitious pacing. "They always feel great initially," explains Gregory Blain, one of Amann's colleagues. "They're flying. But we know they're going to crash." After a blissfully fast start, the nerve-blocked cyclists start to slow down. By the halfway mark, they still feel great, but they start to look puzzled, because their legs are no longer responding to the signals from their brain. They've unwittingly pushed hard enough that the muscles themselves are failing (a topic we'll explore in more detail, along with some other implications of Amann's work, in the next chapter). Without pain, in other words, they're incapable of pacing themselves.

It's tempting to leave the story there, as a tidy Goldilocks tale where a little bit of pain helps pace you but too much slows you down. But as the role of pain in endurance exercise has attracted more research attention, the tale has taken some unexpected turns. In 2013, Alexis Mauger, who had led the first Tylenol study along with several follow-up studies on the topic, took to the online journal *Frontiers in Physiology* with a call to action. Fatigue is often studied in the lab using "time-to-exhaustion" tests, in which the pace or power output is fixed and the subject rides or runs until he or she gives up. But in the real world, Mauger argued, we don't just run to the point of failure; we pace ourselves to go as fast as possible *while never reaching failure.* This process of managing fatigue over a prolonged period of time— enduring the rack rather than submitting to the guillotine—puts a greater emphasis on managing pain. It's no coincidence, then, that pain "is frequently referred to by athletes, coaches and commentators, but has received peculiarly little focus in research," he wrote.

To correct this oversight, Mauger called for more research into the "fatigue-pain relationship"—and in particular for the use of "novel neurophysiological techniques" to modify pain. The reason: even seemingly clear-cut studies like his Tylenol experiment can be interpreted in different ways. Tylenol, after all, fights fever in addition to dulling pain. Could its endurance boosting benefits result from its ability to help prevent your core from overheating, rather than from its pain-blocking effects? It's impossible to be sure.

Taking his own advice, Mauger started experimenting with other ways of altering pain. In one trial, he tried two different ways of applying electric current directly to muscles: transcutaneous electric nerve stimulation (TENS), and interferential current (IFC). Both tools are familiar sights in physical therapy clinics; neither is backed by particularly robust evidence. Their pain-blocking powers rely on the "gate control" theory of pain, which was first proposed in the 1960s. If you whack your shin against a chair, your first instinct will be to rub your bruised shin with your hand. Why? Because the nonpainful sensation of rubbing competes with the pain of the bruise for the same neural signaling pathways that report back to your brain. The more you rub, the less bandwidth is left for pain signals. TENS and IFC are, in effect, a hyperefficient form of rubbing, designed to trigger nonpainful nerve signals that crowd out the painful ones.

At a 2015 conference on endurance research at the University of Kent (where Mauger now works in the Endurance Research Group), he presented his initial findings. To almost everyone's surprise—"I really wasn't expecting anything in particular to happen, to be honest," Mauger admitted—both TENS and IFC, administered to the biceps, significantly improved time to exhaustion among volunteers sustaining an arm-muscle contraction, while a sham trial with no current didn't. "One of the really interesting things about this study," Mauger added, "was that we didn't find any change in RPE [rating of perceived exertion]." Untangling the sensations of pain and effort during exercise, which most of us think of interchangeably, has proven to be remarkably difficult—but in this case, the improvement in endurance seemed clearly linked to suppression of pain rather than effort.

As you might guess from the discussion in Chapter 4, Samuele Marcora, Mauger's colleague at the University of Kent, holds a different view of the relative importance of pain compared to effort. At the same conference, Marcora presented his own data on the primacy of effort. First, to establish the range of possible pain, he and his colleagues Walter Staiano and John Parkinson asked volunteers to complete a "cold pressor" test, a standard protocol used in pain research (such as Wolfgang Freund's study of ultra-runners, discussed above): You dip your hand in a bucket of ice water and hold it there as long as possible, while periodically rating your pain on a scale of 0 to 10. Typically, the pain mounts steadily until you reach an unbearable 10, then you quit.

With this experience of maximal pain fresh in their minds, the subjects then completed a time-to-exhaustion cycling test at a moderately hard pace. During the test, they again rated pain on the 0 to 10 scale, and they also rated effort using Borg's 6-to-20 scale. When the cyclists reached exhaustion, after about 12 minutes, their pain ratings averaged 4.8, corresponding to moderate pain. Their effort ratings, on the other hand, averaged 19.6, which is pretty much as high as it goes. In this context, then, it appears to be effort rather than pain that calls the shots.

So how do you reconcile these seemingly conflicting results? First, you have to make sure you're talking about the same thing when you use the word *pain*. To that end, Mauger and Marcora teamed up to try out a form of electric brain stimulation called tDCS (transcranial direct-current stimulation), which involves running a weak current directly through the various regions of the brain to change the excitability of neurons. The potential of tDCS to enhance learning, mood, motor function, and even (as we'll see in Chapter 11) endurance has earned it a wave of hype in recent years. When directed at the brain's motor cortex, it also has pain-suppressing properties, which is what Mauger and Marcora were interested in here.

They ran two parallel tDCS experiments: the first was an all-out cycling test to exhaustion, and the second was an eight-minute cold pressor test. In both cases, subjects completed each test three times: once with real tDCS, once with sham tDCS with no electric current, and once with no intervention. In the cold pressor test, brain stimulation resulted in lower pain ratings right from the start, and the final pain ratings were, on average, a point lower (7.4 versus 8.4 in the sham trial and 8.6 in the control trial). But in the cycling test, the pain scores were identical in all three trials. The results suggested that the pain you experience in the extremes of sustained exercise is fundamentally different, from your brain's perspective, from the pain you experience while dunking your hand in ice water. All pleasure is alike, as Leo Tolstoy might have put it, but each pain hurts in its own unique way.

The doors to the Velodrome Suisse in Grenchen, a small town midway between Zurich and Geneva, opened at 5:30 P.M. on September 18, 2014. The time had been precisely calculated to allow the collective presence of 1,600 fans to warm and humidify the air in the building to just the right degree before the start of Voigt's record attempt, 90 minutes later: warm air is less dense and thus offers an aerodynamic advantage, but too much warmth risks overheating the cyclist. These were the kinds of details that Voigt's team had fretted endlessly over, and the result of all this careful preparation was that he knew he was capable of the record—but he also knew how slender his margin of error was: "You can have a puncture. You can start out too fast. You can just have a bad day. Hey, you can even have two punctures."

These were the thoughts caroming around in Voigt's mind as—with the help of two assistants—he wriggled into a specially designed, sausage-tight skin suit in the locker room. With a packed stadium, more than four million cycling fans around the world watching him on television, and others tuning in to the live Internet stream, it's easy to understand why he felt acutely anxious in these final minutes. And yet for a man about to test the limits of his own pain tolerance for a full hour, this was a crucial advantage. Like a wounded soldier on a battlefield, or a kudu cornered by a hungry lion, athletes in the heat of competition exhibit a phenomenon called "stress-induced analgesia," which enables them to ignore otherwise debilitating levels of pain. Finally, the starting gun fired, and, to the technopunk beat of Republica's mid-1990s hit "Ready to Go," Voigt stood up in his saddle and began pedaling.

Some of the most epic tales and Bunyanesque feats in sports involve athletes who defied pain to score the winning point or outlast their opponent: hockey player Bobby Baun's overtime winner for the Toronto Maple Leafs in the 1964 Stanley Cup Finals, skating on an ankle he had fractured earlier in the game; Willis Reed taking on Wilt Chamberlain in the 1970 NBA Finals with a torn thigh muscle; Kerri Strug's gold-medal-clinching vault on a sprained ankle at the 1996 Olympics. In fact, playing through a broken limb isn't even that rare, even when the stakes are lower: Philadelphia Eagles quarterback Donovan McNabb had the best passing game of his career on a broken ankle in 2002; Boston Bruins center Gregory Campbell played out a shorthanded shift after a slap shot broke his fibula during the 2013 playoffs; Denver Broncos safety David Bruton Jr. played another ninety-five snaps on a broken fibula after a first-quarter collision in 2015.

And it's not just bruisers in full-contact sports who do it. At the Vancouver Olympics in 2010, Slovenian cross-country skier Petra Majdič slipped during her warm-up and fell ten feet into a rock-strewn creek. Not realizing that she had broken five ribs, she skied through excruciating pain in her qualifying round, quarterfinals, semifinals (during which one of the cracked ribs pierced a lung, causing it to collapse), and finals, where she earned a stupendously improbable bronze medal. Then, finally, she went to the hospital.

There's no doubt these athletes are tough. But their heroics are also, to some extent, enabled by the circumstances. The way most of us think of pain was most famously articulated by French philosopher René Descartes in his 1664 *Treatise of Man:* you whack your thumb with a hammer, and this sends a message that, in Descartes's imagery, rings a bell in your brain. In this view, there's a one-to-one correspondence between the damage or injury you've suffered and the pain you feel. The problem with this view is that the same injury can provoke dramatically different reactions in different people, or even in the same person at different times. At the opposite extreme, amputees with phantom limb syndrome experience real pain that has no physical source.

As a result, starting with observations of wounded soldiers during the U.S. Civil War, doctors and pain researchers have concluded that pain is fundamentally a subjective, situation-dependent phenomenon.

For example, stress, fear, and anxiety activate an impressive array of brain chemicals, including endorphins (the body's store-brand opioid drugs) and endocannabinoids (the body's cannabis), to dull or completely block pain that would overwhelm you in other circumstances. In evolutionary terms, pain may serve a valuable function by telling you to stop and allow an injury to heal. "But if you're a deer being chased by a wolf and you trip and break a leg," says Mogil, the McGill pain researcher, "you need to forget about that pain until later."

Breaking your leg and chasing a new marathon best, it should be said, differ greatly in the nature and degree of pain incurred. The palette of pain is infinitely variable, and athletes sample widely. Even without broken ribs, a sprint skier like Majdič, whose event lasts less than four minutes, will encounter a flood of metabolites that sear her muscles from within. An ultra-runner might run for hours at a seemingly easy pace but eventually be hobbled by cumulative microtears in her muscles that send high-voltage bursts of pain through her calves and quads with every step. And somewhere between these two extremes—the worst of both worlds, according to those who have tried it—lies the Hour.

Part of the Hour's horror lies in its setting: no scenery, no competitors, no pace changes, almost no external feedback of any sort. The lack of distraction robs you of a powerful way of altering how the brain perceives pain, the psychological version of rubbing a bruise to interfere with pain signals in the muscle. But the duration of the race also happens to lie on a physiological knife edge. There are many ways of delineating the boundary between short and uncomfortable high-intensity exercise and longer, more pleasant efforts. One of the most familiar is *lactate threshold,* the point at which you're working hard enough that levels of lactate in your blood start creeping inexorably upward. A more recently developed concept is *critical power,* which is the point beyond which your muscles can no longer stay in the sustainable "steady state" equilibrium fetishized by Harvard Fatigue Laboratory researchers. Sixty minutes of all-out exercise, for a well-trained athlete, sits in the excruciating gap between these two markers, explains Mark Burnley, a physiologist in the University of Kent's Endurance Research Group. "Riders in the Hour have to exercise above lactate threshold, but very slightly below the critical power—in other words, ride with the highest metabolic rate that is also steady state." Done right, then, the Hour is literally the longest bout of painful high-intensity exercise you can endure.

For Voigt's final professional ride—the king of pain attacking the sport's ultimate test of mental mettle—the most painful challenge turned out to be saddle sores from the awkward and unfamiliar riding position. He had started quickly, covering the 250-meter laps in just over 17 seconds, and soon built a comfortable margin ahead of his pre-ride goal of averaging 17.9 seconds per lap. The first 10 minutes felt easy; after 20 minutes, as the fatigue set in, he throttled back slightly, searching for that knife edge of sustainability. By the halfway point, his tailbones were so raw that he began to stand up out of the saddle every ten laps to relieve the pressure—a flagrant aerodynamic faux-pas for a rider whose sponsors had provided a special skin suit, wind-defying gloves, and even drag-minimizing socks.

In this case, Voigt was far enough ahead of the record that his saddle sores didn't scuttle the effort. By the time he passed two hundred laps, the triumphant synth of Europe's "The Final Countdown" spurring on his last push, he had the record well enough in hand that he could finally let his thoughts wander briefly. There was pride in his achievement, joy that it had all gone according to plan, relief that it was almost over, all mixed with sadness that his days of stardom were ending. Finally, the gun sounded to signal the Hour's end, and the pain he'd been pushing to the margins of his consciousness came crashing down: "Everything was aching. My neck ached from holding my head low in that aerodynamic position. My elbows hurt from holding my upper body in that position. My lungs hurt after burning and screaming for oxygen for so long. My heart hurt from the constant pounding. My back was on fire, and then there was my butt! I was really and truly in a world of pain."

The scoreboard read 51,110 meters, eclipsing the previous record by 1,410 meters—nearly a mile. Voigt's record lasted all of six weeks before falling to an unheralded Austrian named Matthias Brändle, at twenty-four years old nearly two decades younger than Voigt. The record fell three more times in 2015, the last time to a true heavyweight, former Tour de France winner and five-time Olympic champion Bradley Wiggins, who pushed the record out to 54,526 meters. Voigt's timing, thanks to the confluence of the UCI rule change and his impending retirement, was certainly lucky. But his name is—and will always remain—on one of the most exclusive lists in cycling.

Did Voigt really suffer more than the rest of us? While there are still plenty of gaps in the research, it does appear that top athletes really push themselves to a darker place, and stay there longer, than most people are willing to tolerate. But the more interesting comparison isn't between Voigt and Joe Sixpack; it's between Voigt and Wiggins and the rest of the elite peloton. Studies of truly elite athletes are few and far between, and it's nearly impossible to collect heat-of-the-battle data when the athletes are pushing hardest. Remember Tim Noakes's picture of the Olympic marathon champion and the man he had just outsprinted by three seconds: did the silver medalist really let immortality slip from his grasp because it hurt too much? The experiments that Alexis Mauger and Samuele Marcora have done trying to untangle the difference between "pain" and "effort" make me think that pain, in most contexts, is a warning light on the dashboard. It instructs you (sometimes very insistently) to slow down, and in most contexts you heed that warning without even realizing you're doing it. But it's not an absolute limit. For that, we have to look elsewhere.

CHAPTER 6

Muscle

On a warm Tucson evening in July 2006, Tom Boyle and his wife, Elizabeth, were waiting to merge from a shopping mall parking lot onto South Kolb Road, a fast-moving six-lane thoroughfare. The car in front of their pickup truck, a Camaro, squealed its tires to seize a gap in the passing traffic—and suddenly there was a shower of sparks. "Oh my God," Elizabeth blurted. "Do you see that?" The car had plowed into a cyclist riding the wrong way along South Kolb and was now dragging both rider and bike along the road underneath it. Boyle leapt out of his pickup truck and started running as the Camaro, twenty or thirty feet away, finally slithered to a halt.

You know how this story goes. Boyle found the cyclist, eighteen-year-old Kyle Holtrust, pinned under the front wheels of the car. "As soon as I get to the car, the boy is just screaming his head off, and I could tell he was in a lot of pain," Boyle later recalled. So he lifted the car up. "Mister, mister, higher, higher!" Holtrust screamed. When it was high enough, Boyle yelled to the Camaro's driver, who snapped out of a daze and pulled Holtrust out. Then he put the car down and held Holtrust in his arms until emergency personnel arrived. The boy survived, and Boyle's feat entered the crowded but hard-to-verify annals of "hysterical strength."

When your legs fail you, it's natural to blame your legs. The same is true whether you're lifting a piano, pedaling a bike up the Alpe d'Huez, or clinging by your fingertips to a narrow fissure in an overhanging rock face: there are times when it feels like your muscles are simply and unambiguously maxed out. In prolonged tests of endurance, this feeling is muddied by all the other sensations flooding your synapses—pounding heart, rasping lungs, flagging willpower, and so on. In short, all-out efforts, on the other hand, we get a much cleaner picture: either you can lift the car or you can't. That's why feats like Boyle's are so confounding: in the long-running debate about whether we're able to use every ounce of strength our muscles possess, they seem to demolish everything we think we know.

Muscles do have limits, of course. As far back as the nineteenth century, physiologists were wiring up frog legs and making them dance with electric shocks until the muscles became totally unresponsive. And, in those heady days before universities had research ethics boards, it was a short step to trying similar experiments on humans. Researchers like Angelo Mosso, the Italian physiologist who pioneered the study of mental fatigue (as described in Chapter 4), tried to compare the force his subjects could produce voluntarily with the force their muscles could produce when stimulated electrically. If the involuntary contractions were stronger than the voluntary ones, the thinking went, it would demonstrate that we have some sort of protective mechanism—a central governor for strength, in effect—to make sure we don't tear our tendons and yank our muscles off the bone. But at that point, measurement techniques weren't advanced enough to settle the question one way or the other.

There were, however, other hints of muscular capacity held in reserve. In 1939, for example, German researchers published the results of their experiments with a newly developed drug called Pervitin, showing that endurance in a cycling test could be tripled with no apparent changes in metabolism or circulation. Their conclusion was that "the end point of any performance is never an absolute fixed point but rather is when the sum of all negative factors such as fatigue and muscle pain are felt more strongly than the positive factors of motivation and will power."

The drug was early version of crystal methamphetamine, and German military officials took a keen interest in the results. They piloted Pervitin later that year on military drivers deployed in the invasion of

Poland, which triggered World War II; convinced of its usefulness, the Nazis distributed it to all branches of the military. Between April and July 1940 alone, more than 35 million tablets of "Panzerschokolade" (tank chocolate) fueled the Blitzkrieg across Europe, spurring lasting rumors of a Nazi superpill that gave soldiers extraordinary powers. (The dark aftereffects of crystal meth became clearer over time, and German officials restricted its used in 1941, though it remained widely used until the end of the war—and stayed part of the East German army's war chest until 1988.)

Tom Boyle wasn't on crystal meth when he lifted the car, but he certainly had adrenaline coursing through his veins. In a series of experiments in the late 1950s, researchers Michio Ikai (a former student of A. V. Hill) and Arthur Steinhaus tested some of the ways that extreme situations like near-death experiences might enhance strength. They instructed their subjects to flex their forearms as hard as possible once per minute, each time the second hand of an electric timer swept past one o'clock, for thirty minutes. Injections of adrenaline, they reported in the *Journal of Applied Physiology*, produced a statistically insignificant increase of 6.5 percent in strength; amphetamine tablets boosted strength more robustly, by 13.5 percent. Better yet, having one of the researchers, "standing directly behind the unwarned subject," fire a .22-caliber starter's gun a few seconds before a scheduled contraction boosted the strength of that contraction by an average of 7.4 percent.

These results are often trotted out as evidence that feats of superhuman strength are possible under the right circumstances. What's seldom mentioned is that Ikai and Steinhaus also claimed to see average strength increases of 26.5 percent after hypnosis, with large increases persisting even after the hypnotic state was broken. The power of these trances was so great that when the hypnotist touched one skeptical subject with a fountain pen, while telling him that it was a red-hot poker, "the blister that appeared within the hour took a week to heal and served to convince the subject of the reality of hypnosis."

The increases in strength, the researchers argued, occurred because hypnosis (or drugs or fright) allowed the subjects to overcome their deep-seated inhibitions. For example, one "athletically inclined, yet genuinely feminine" subject had as a child been constantly warned by her mother not to overdo exertion, and was mocked and called "Miss Football" in high school for being too athletic. Hypnosis, according to Ikai and Steinhaus, allowed her to leave the resulting inhibitions behind and increase her strength by 50 percent. It's worth noting that, more than half a century later, these findings haven't been replicated under controlled conditions.

There's also a key difference between lifting a car once, and producing "maximal" contractions over and over again. In 2014, a team led by Israel Halperin at Memorial University of Newfoundland tried a similar experiment, with subjects doing five-second maximal biceps curls (against an immovable resistance) every 15 seconds. One group was told they'd be doing 6 contractions; another was told they'd be doing 12; and a third group was simply told to keep going until instructed to stop. But once the experiment started, all three groups had to do 12. In theory, the instructions shouldn't have made any difference, because the subjects were explicitly and repeatedly told *not* to pace themselves: each contraction was supposed to be as hard as possible, with nothing held in reserve.

In practice, though, expectations mattered. Within a few reps, those who thought they were only doing 6 were producing slightly more force than the 12-rep control group; and those with no information about how long they would be expected to continue were producing less force than the other groups. Not surprisingly, the average force declined with each succeeding rep—until the last one (and the sixth one, in the deceived group), when they were able to summon a "finishing kick" to exert more force. The pattern, overall, looked a lot like the U-shaped pattern observed in distance-running world records (see page 49), and like my own hardwired fast-finish pacing in 5,000-meter races. Even in short, supposedly all-out maximal contractions, when we're explicitly told to hold nothing in reserve, we pace ourselves—

a finding that helps explain why Ikai and Steinhaus were seemingly able to tap into hidden reserves of strength, but doesn't explain how a human can lift a car.

At the 1983 World's Strongest Man competition, in Christchurch, New Zealand, a fresh-faced Canadian powerlifter named Tom Magee (later known as MegaMan during a brief World Wrestling Federation career) deadlifted 1,180 pounds of local cheddar cheese—"enough," the television commentator deadpanned, "to fill an awful lot of mouse-traps." That feat, with two towering stacks of cheese blocks connected by a flexible bar that started eighteen inches off the ground, remains the heaviest verified deadlift on record; the records using standard bars and plates are a bit lighter. In contrast, a typical Camaro, even stripped down for drag racing, weighs at least 3,000 pounds. Even if we assume that life-or-death situations can summon extra strength, that still seems like an awfully large gap.

One commonly cited estimate of the difference between voluntary and truly maximal strength comes from Vladimir Zatsiorsky, a bio-mechanics expert who spent three decades at the Central Institute of Physical Culture in Moscow, the hub of scientific research for the Soviet sport system, before moving to Penn State in the early 1990s. In his 1995 treatise, *Science and Practice of Strength Training,* a dense training bible that still has a cult following, Zatsiorsky reported that most of us can summon about 65 percent of our theoretical maximum strength. Elite weightlifters can do better, hefting more than 80 percent of their maximum in workouts—and with the psychological boost of a big competition, they can lift, according to one of Zatsiorsky's studies, an additional 12.5 percent compared to their training best. Plug these numbers in and you find that Magee, with the fear of God buzzing in his circuits, might have been able to hoist another one or two hundred pounds of cheese—but still less than half a Camaro.

So how did Zatsiorsky determine the "true" maximum strength of his weightlifters? That is either lost in the mists of time or buried in obscure mid-twentieth-century Soviet sports journals. Some experts are highly skeptical: Guillaume Millet, a French researcher who heads the University of Calgary's Neuromuscular Fatigue Lab, says Zatsiorsky's numbers are "absolutely crazy." When I contacted Zatsiorsky in 2016, he was eighty-three years old, long retired from Penn State, but still very active as a researcher—he was listed as coauthor of no less than seven academic journal articles dealing with the subtleties of motor control that were published between January and September of that year. But he couldn't fill in any details about his much-quoted maximum strength numbers. "Unfortunately," he told me in an email, "I do not remember who mentioned these facts first." That doesn't automatically mean they're wrong—after all, one of the reasons they crop up in so many "scientific explanations" of superhuman strength is that they sound plausible. But plausibility isn't the same as proof.

While no one has managed to definitively confirm or refute Zatsiorsky's findings, it's not for lack of trying. The idea that we all harbor a hidden reserve of muscular strength gained currency in the early 1900s as experiments with electricity proliferated: as a pair of Danish researchers wrote in 1923, "everyone who has experience of having his muscles stimulated by electrical stimuli knows that it is possible in this way to obtain contractions of a force which is quite impossible to reproduce voluntarily." But actually measuring this reserve was challenging, because most human movements use several different muscle groups triggered by different nerve pathways, unlike the crude single-muscle twitch produced by an electric shock.

It wasn't until 1954 that a cheerfully eccentric British physiologist named Patrick Merton devised a solution. He would clamp a subject's forearm—usually his own, leaving the other hand free to take measurements—so that only the thumb could move, and only in one specific direction activated by the adductor pollicis muscle. When he compared the thumb's maximal voluntary force with the force produced by an escalating series of sustained electric shocks to the associated nerve, repeated up to fifty times per second, he came to two surprising conclusions. First, the force produced by the shocks *felt* far greater. (They also hurt: "The considerable pain caused is minimized if the skin under the stimulating electrode is not broken," he noted.) And second, the actual force was essentially the same. The supposed reserve of muscular strength, in other words, was an illusion—a result, Merton concluded, that flew in the face of the then-widespread belief that "lunatics, persons suffering from tetanus or convulsions or under hypnosis, and those drowning are exceptionally powerful."

Merton strengthened his case with a novel twist. While his subjects voluntarily contracted their thumb muscles, he superimposed a brief electrical twitch. If the voluntary contraction was relatively weak, the force would jump significantly when the twitch was added; but for stronger voluntary contractions, the size of the twitch got progressively smaller. And for maximal contractions, the brief electric shock didn't add any force at all, suggesting once again that no extra muscle remained unused.

In the years since then, similar experiments have been repeated many times under many different conditions. In addition to triggering muscle contractions with electric shocks, researchers now use pulses of magnetic stimulation directly to the brain's motor cortex to produce short muscle contractions elsewhere in the body (another technique pioneered, using more painful electric shocks to his own skull, by the intrepid Merton), in order to tease out where and how fatigue takes place. Overall, according to Roger Enoka, who directs the University of Colorado Boulder's Neurophysiology of Movement Lab, the modern consensus from these studies echoes Merton's finding: most healthy people can achieve "voluntary action scores" of close to 100 percent. In Mark Burnley's lab, at the University of Kent, typical scores for all-out quadriceps contractions are 92 to 97 percent, and anything less than 90 percent suggests something has gone wrong with the test. Under normal conditions, in other words, we're utilizing pretty much all the strength our muscles have to offer.

There are, however, two possible loopholes, Enoka notes. One is that you can't sustain 100 percent activation indefinitely, so the idea of a hidden muscle reserve makes more sense for cyclists and rowers and runners than for piano movers. The other is the difference between twitching your thumb and, say, deadlifting a car—a movement that requires a deceptively intricate synchronized pattern of activation involving at least thirteen different muscle groups. It's possible that these complex real-world actions make it harder to reach full voluntary activation in all the relevant muscle groups, meaning there might be some reserve accessible in stressful situations. This prospect hasn't been tested, Enoka says, and it's not clear that such a test is even possible with current technology (which is why Zatsiorsky's claims are so intriguing).

With this loophole in mind, Tom Boyle's Camaro-hoisting exploits remain at least plausible—especially when you factor in some basic but often-neglected physics. Boyle, after all, didn't lift the car right off the ground. At most, he raised the front axle, which would involve lifting less than half the weight of the car, thanks to the leverage advantage provided by lifting from the very front. But even that may be an overestimate, thanks to the car's suspension system. Think about what happens when you change a spare tire: the jack lifts only one wheel off the ground, elevating (at a very rough estimate) a quarter of the car's weight, which for a Camaro is in the range of 750 pounds. And Boyle may not have needed to actually get the front wheel (or wheels) airborne to free the cyclist; he just had to get enough weight off the victim to allow the driver of the car to pull the cyclist out from underneath.

Without seeing the exact details of the rescue, it's impossible to know how much force the feat required. But 800 pounds could conceivably have been enough. And Boyle is (as journalist Jeff Wise described him) "no pantywaist": he's 6'4", weighs 280 pounds, and has deadlifted 700 pounds in the gym. Add in Zatsiorsky's 20 percent reserve for experienced weightlifters and you get a potential "true strength" of 840 pounds. Of the many stories of superhuman strength out there, this one comes closest to passing the sniff test. Whatever happened that night, it seems clear the horror of the situation allowed Boyle to transcend his normal limits: it wasn't until he got home that

night that he noticed he had clenched his jaw so tightly during the lift
that he had broken eight teeth.

By the time Stéphane Couleaud reached the alpine town of Donnas,
he had been running for almost 34 hours. He had traversed 95 miles
of vertiginous trails across the peaks and passes encircling the Valle
d'Aosta, the valley on the Italian side of the point where the Italian,
French, and Swiss borders collide, alternately shivering and sweating
as he passed in and out of cold rains and valley microclimates and the
sun rose, set, and rose again. The route had taken him up (and down)
more than 35,000 feet—an Everest and a quarter. And he wasn't even
halfway done.

Couleaud, an experienced mountain runner who in 2009 had set
a record with a ten-day traverse of the Pyrenees, was sitting in sev-
enth place in one of the most grueling ultra-trail races in the world,
the Tor des Géants. By the admittedly warped standards of the ultra-
endurance world, the race's 205-mile distance is relatively tame. (You
want crazy? Try a double deca Ironman triathlon, which starts with
a 47-mile swim, followed by a 2,200-mile bike ride and a 524-mile
run, and takes about 20 days to finish . . . if you're the winner.) But
the race's punishing topography, with ankle-twisting trails and nearly
80,000 feet of ascent and descent as it skirts four of the tallest mountains in the Alps (Mont Blanc, Gran Paradiso, Monte Rosa, and the
Matterhorn), is what sets it apart. With no scheduled rest breaks, the
top runners typically complete the course in around 80 hours, pausing for at most a few hours of sleep. If there is a race that will squeeze
every last twitch from your aching quads, this is the one.

In the aid station at Donnas, Couleaud paused to refuel and take
a short break—but first, a pair of researchers rushed him through a
thirty-minute sequence of tests. His body composition was measured
with a ZMetrix bioimpedance system; a nurse drew blood and measured the circumference of his thighs and calves to check for inflammation; he whizzed through a computerized cognitive test; he completed

a series of maximal leg contractions, with and without electrical stimulation, to assess the decline in muscle strength and voluntary activation; and he balanced, first with eyes open then with eyes closed, on a force-measuring plate—until, as his body struggled to adjust its blood pressure to the luxury of rest, he passed out. He had completed the same tests before the race started, and would complete them again at the finish—if he made it.

One of the masterminds behind this cruel ordeal was Guillaume Millet, who in addition to his research role was a former national-team cross-country skier and accomplished ultra-trail runner: he had finished third in the 2010 Tor des Géants. For more than a decade, Millet had been studying muscle fatigue at the opposite end of the spectrum from Merton's short maximal spasms, trying to quantify and explain the loss of force in progressively longer and more extreme challenges—a ski marathon, a five-hour treadmill run, a twenty-four-hour treadmill run, the 100-mile Ultra Trail Mont-Blanc, and now the 2011 Tor des Géants. (The Tor des Géants study was, as it happens, coordinated by Guillaume's brother Grégoire, a sports physiologist at the University of Lausanne who went on to surpass Guillaume's accomplishment by finishing second in the race in 2012.)

The basic measure of fatigue Guillaume Millet uses in his studies is simple: how much does the biggest force you can produce with a given muscle decline? Not surprisingly, he has found that the force produced by two key muscle groups in the legs, the quadriceps and the calves, gets progressively weaker as the distance of a running race increases—up to a point. By the time you've been out there for about 24 hours, your leg muscles will be 35 to 40 percent weaker, and they won't lose much more. In fact, his Tor des Géants subjects, who took more than 100 hours, on average, to complete the race, ended up losing just 25 percent of their pre-race leg strength—a result that, on the surface, makes little sense. "Okay," Millet jokes, "so if I run 200 miles, I'm less fatigued than if I run 100 miles!"

This counterintuitive finding, on its own, already hints that leg muscles aren't what ultimately limit ultra-endurance athletes. And there are some more subtle details. The electrically stimulated twitch data allows Millet to estimate how much of the force loss is due to fatigue in the muscles themselves, and how much is "central," reflecting either diminished output from the brain or losses in transmission via the spinal cord. For ultra-endurance runs, it turns out, the muscles themselves typically only lose about 10 percent of their force-producing capacity; the rest is central, reflecting a progressive decline in the brain's voluntary activation of muscle. "The brain is able to do more, but it doesn't," Millet says. But, he adds, that doesn't necessarily mean the brain is *responsible* for this decline.

When Millet compared muscle fatigue following three hours of running to similar durations of cycling and cross-country skiing, he found that voluntary activation declined by 8 percent in running but didn't change in cycling or skiing. The difference between these three activities? The impact forces in running cause microscopic damage that alters the properties of your leg muscles, unlike the two impact-free activities. Even though voluntary activation is, by definition, a reduction in the command signal from your brain, it appears to respond to what's happening in your muscles. We have special nerve fibers that send information from the muscles to the brain about pressure, heat, damage, metabolic disturbances, and any number of other data points, and we integrate this information in our actions without even realizing it. Trying to make a clean divide between "brain fatigue" and "muscle fatigue," in other words, is inevitably an oversimplification, because they're inseparably linked.

Perhaps more important, the link between leg fatigue—whether central or peripheral—and actual race performance is far from straightforward. "Okay, so I'm losing 40 percent of my maximal force," Millet says. "Is that the explanation for why my speed is reduced? No . . . at least not directly." If you're competing in a 100-mile race, the pace you'll be running at the 95-mile mark will require far less than 60 percent of your maximal muscle output. If a bear jumps out from behind a tree, you will discover you can still sprint—which means that, whatever was dictating your pace, it wasn't the inability of your muscles to deliver more force. That's the same observation that Samuele Marcora made in his 2010 "mind over muscle" study (described on page 60): his subjects cycled at 242 watts until they could no longer continue, but were somehow able to generate 731 watts in a five-second sprint. At the point of exhaustion in a long endurance challenge, the legs are merely unwilling, not incapable.

So if it's not muscle fatigue, what is it? Both Marcora and Millet argue that a variety of factors feed into the brain's decision to speed up, slow down, or stop. In ultra-races like the Tor des Géants, relatively unsexy talents like the ability to scarf down prodigious amounts of calorie-rich food and keep running without throwing up are absolutely crucial. If you can't do that, an empty fuel tank will be your limiting factor. In hilly mountain races, the microscopic muscle damage inflicted with each stride is magnified by the jarring eccentric muscle contractions as you race downhill (a drama that plays out in miniature in the early downhill miles of the Boston Marathon every April). If your legs aren't hardened against the rigors of downhill running, your muscles really will limit your speed—but as a result of structural damage, and the associated pain and loss of coordination, rather than ordinary fatigue.

For Stéphane Couleaud, these and many other factors were coming together perfectly during the second half of the race—no blisters, no stomach problems, and his legs continued to carry him up and down the mountain trails without complaint. By the time he stopped for three minutes to down a beer and some solid food at the alpine hut below the 9,000-foot Champillon col, he had moved up to fourth place and was more than 12 hours ahead of his pace from the previous year. The trouble, when it came, seemed minor at first: he felt too hot. In the village of Bosses, he stripped off his T-shirt, shorts, and shoes and jumped into a fountain to cool off for five minutes. Back on the trail, he pressed on as night fell. A text message arrived telling him that one of the runners ahead of him was disqualified, moving him up to third. The news buoyed him but also filled him with a sense of urgency, and he hurried on despite flashes of dizziness and overheating.

By that point, he recalls, "I knew I was failing." During the descent to the penultimate hut, just seven miles from the finish—a section of the trail he knew by heart—he lost his way five times. And when he arrived, he made a catastrophically bad decision, waving off the meal, hot drink, and bed offered by the hut keeper and plunging back into the night after downing a glass of water, without even refilling his bottles. "I was unable to think and reason," he says. "My brain did not work correctly."

Fifteen minutes later, he collapsed. He had been running for 85 hours and 30 minutes, stopping to rest for a total of just 3 hours and 20 minutes. Millet, in his own race a year earlier, had done something similar—less than 3 hours of sleep during an 87-hour effort—and was hallucinating by the end, unable to distinguish between waking and dreaming. Couleaud wasn't so lucky—though the weather, mild by mountain standards, was fortunate indeed. Although his legs would no longer carry him, he managed to wrap himself in his feather-light emergency blanket without tearing it and turn his headlamp to flashing mode, then dialed Millet on his cell phone. It was after midnight, so Millet had already turned his phone off. "When I got the message the following morning, I thought he was dead," Millet recalls. "The message was hardly audible, like someone dying." Ninety minutes later, another runner arrived and wrapped Couleaud in his Gore-Tex vest and another emergency blanket. Eventually, Couleaud woke to a violent shaking from a doctor accompanied by a mountain guide; they took him down to their four-by-four a half-hour hike away, and then back to civilization.

"We are rarely running to death," Millet says. Factors like excessive heat, drugs, and prolonged sleep deprivation—the likely culprit in Couleaud's ordeal—can alter the body's delicate balance, but "our brain protects us against our own excess—almost always."

Most of life, of course, plays out somewhere between the extremes—neither lifting a car nor running through the mountains for eighty hours straight. So where is the crossover between short, muscle-limited acts of strength and prolonged tests of will? To explore this question, Norwegian researcher Christian Frøyd, working under the joint supervision of Guillaume Millet and Tim Noakes, put volunteers through a series of time trials lasting 3, 10, and 40 minutes. The "time trials" were a little unusual—instead of the typical exercise bike or treadmill, the subjects had to forcefully kick their legs once every two seconds while strapped into a force-measuring device called a dynamometer. The advantage of this setup was that the apparatus permitted tests of maximum voluntary force, with or without an additional electric shock, as frequently as every minute. Since muscles begin recovering from fatigue within a few seconds, this is the only way to get reliable fatigue measurements that aren't skewed by the time it takes to get off a bike and into a dynamometer.

The results, which were published in 2016, echoed some of the patterns in Millet's ultra-endurance data: muscle fatigue dominated in the shortest trials, while central fatigue was increasingly important in the longer ones. In fact, the maximal force measurements taken during the longer trials showed that fatigue in the muscles themselves soon reached a fairly stable plateau at about 80 percent of full strength, which persisted until the subjects launched into their finishing kick at the end of the trial. That suggests that the importance of purely muscle-based fatigue in long events has been, if anything, *over*estimated by previous studies. If your leg muscles are really shot at the end of a one-hour race, it's largely because you high-stepped down the final straightaway.

The most interesting detail in Frøyd's study is the pacing. In the 10- and 40-minute trials, just as in the mile, 5,000- and 10,000-meter running world records plotted in the graph on page 49, the subjects sped up to finish with a flourish. In the three-minute trial, on the other hand, they struggled to simply avoid slowing down too much—which, not coincidentally, is the near-ironclad rule in 800-meter racing, as the same graph shows.

When David Rudisha, a long, lean twenty-three-year-old from the

Masai tribe in Kenya, set the current 800-meter record of 1:40.91 at the 2012 London Olympics, he ran his first lap in 49.28 seconds and his second lap in 51.63 seconds—a slowdown of 2.35 seconds. That's typical of elite 800-meter races, according to Ross Tucker's analysis of world-record pacing: in all records going back to the first modern record in 1912, the second lap has been on average 2.4 seconds slower than the first lap. Only twice in that time has an 800-meter record been set with a faster second lap, which is the opposite of what is seen in longer races. In fact, the three-second improvement in the record since the 1960s is almost entirely due to runners speeding through a faster first lap; the second lap has stayed nearly constant, suggesting some sort of physiological limit for sprinting on fatigued legs.

Such patterns are highly unlikely to occur purely by chance, and Frøyd's data offers some clues about what is going on. He put electrodes on his subjects' quadriceps muscles to measure the electrical impulses passing from the brain to the muscle, as a way of approximating how strongly the brain was demanding contractions. In the 10- and 40-minute trials, these EMG signals mirrored the actual force produced by the muscles, with a sharp increase in both EMG and force near the end of the trials. But in the three-minute trials, the patterns were different: while the force was gradually decreasing, the EMG signal was still increasing. In a three-minute trial (and presumably in 800-meter races), the brain still calls for a sprint as the finish line approaches; the muscles are simply unable to obey. If you're looking for the midpoint between the muscle's role in hoisting a car and the brain's role in running an ultra, this is as good a definition as any: that agonizing point, about 600 meters into an 800-meter race, where you're holding nothing back but can feel yourself slowing anyway.

Runners have a phrase for that feeling, though it doesn't show up in dictionaries: to rig, as in "I thought I was going to win the race, but I started rigging on the final turn." It's derived from *rigor mortis,* the stiffening of the body after death, and it's one of those words that perfectly capture an otherwise baffling sensation. Sometimes, when you're watching a middle-distance race, you can see the exact moment when someone starts tying up (another euphemism in common use), as their stride shortens and their movements get jerky—and, if you've been in that situation yourself, you can't help wincing in sympathy.

So why is it that your muscles fail you when you rig? The traditional explanation has long been that they are overwhelmed by a flood of lactic acid, which is produced when you're working so hard that oxygen-fueled aerobic energy supplies can't keep up with demand. After all, rigging typically occurs in events lasting between about one and ten minutes, which corresponds to the duration in which the highest levels of lactate are produced in your blood. And the severity of the rig can be diminished ever so slightly by ingesting baking soda, which counters rising acidity in much the same way that it reacts with acetic acid (that is, vinegar) in grade-school volcano models. (The downside of baking soda doping, while we're on the volcano theme, is the potential for explosive diarrhea.)

While this perception of the "lactic burn" is still widespread, lactate has undergone a rehabilitation in scientific circles thanks primarily to George Brooks, a researcher at the University of California, Berkeley. Brooks and others have shown that lactate plays a complex role in muscles, serving as a crucial source of emergency fuel during intense exercise. Top athletes, far from being immune to lactate, are actually able to recycle it into fuel more efficiently than lesser athletes. Moreover, if lactate was really the problem, you'd be able to reproduce the sensation of rigging by injecting lactate into your muscles—but, as it turns out, it's not that simple.

In a 2014 study, Markus Amann and Alan Light, along with colleagues at the University of Utah, tried injecting three different metabolites associated with intense exercise—lactate, protons, and adenosine triphosphate, or ATP—into the thumb muscles of ten lucky volunteers. The concentrations they used varied from the "normal" concentrations that are always circulating in the body to the higher levels associated with moderate, vigorous, and extreme exercise. On their own, none of the three metabolites had any discernible effect. The same was true when they were injected in pairs, despite the fact that lactate plus protons is what makes lactic acid.

But when they injected all three metabolites together, the volunteers suddenly had the bizarre sensation of extreme fatigue and discomfort—concentrated in their thumbs. At low doses, the sensations reported by the volunteers were mostly things like "tired" and "pressure"; as the doses increased, the sensations ramped up in intensity and shifted to pain-related words like "ache" and "hot." The results suggest that lactic burn isn't literally the feeling of acid dissolving your muscles; instead, it's a cautionary signal created in the brain by nerve endings that are triggered only in the presence of three key metabolites.

As we saw in the previous chapter, Amann has used fentanyl to block these nerve signals, so that his subjects are incapable of feeling this lactate-proton-ATP burn. The result, in cycling time trials, is that the subjects start fast and initially feel great, but eventually run into trouble as their muscles stop responding properly. Amann's theory is that the lactate-proton-ATP feedback is the brain's way of ensuring that the muscles themselves never exceed a critical level of stress and disruption. If you disable this protective system, for example with fentanyl, then you become capable of pushing your muscles closer to their real limits. At that point, elevated levels of other metabolites such as phosphate begin to interfere directly with the ability of muscle fibers to contract.

Is it possible to reach those true muscular limits without fentanyl? In a short all-out sprint of less than a minute or so, undoubtedly. The second-lap plateau in world-class 800-meter runners looks to me like a sign that these runners, too, are smacking into non-negotiable muscular limits—just as, conversely, the fast finish that shows up in races lasting more than two minutes looks like evidence that the brain is in control in these longer events. Are there any exceptions? Under the right circumstances, can you push your muscles to the edge even in a prolonged test of endurance? It probably won't happen in an exercise physiology lab, and perhaps not even in the greatest sporting competitions—but that doesn't mean it's impossible.

In 2012, *Sports Illustrated* writer David Epstein recounted the ordeal of Rhiannon Hull, a talented distance runner who had competed for the University of Oregon's fabled track and cross-country programs. Six weeks after moving to Costa Rica in 2011, she and her six-year-old son, Julian, headed to a local beach on an overcast day when no one else was around, and got pulled away from shore by a riptide. By the time two teenage surfers spotted them and managed to paddle to the rescue, Hull, a wiry 5'2" marathoner who at age thirty-three still ran twice a day, had been holding her son aloft in the water for nearly half an hour—he was "standing on Mommy," he later recalled.

As the two surfers paddled closer, Hull's head was periodically dipping beneath the waves as she struggled to keep Julian up. They arrived just as she launched the boy upward one last time. One of the surfers grabbed Julian and draped him on the surfboard, then turned back to Hull. But she never surfaced again.

It is interesting, if admittedly a bit morbid, to wonder: had no surfers come to rescue her, would she have been able to hold out longer, or would she have succumbed sooner? Either scenario is plausible, and both would indicate that the arrival (or nonarrival) of rescue, like the looming finish line in a race, unlocked a reserve controlled by the brain. But the improbable end of her saga, saving her son but losing herself, makes it tempting to believe that the answer lies balanced exactly in the middle—that after a lifetime of pushing her muscles as close to their limits as possible, Rhiannon Hull finally poured out the full and exact measure of her prodigious endurance.

We will, of course, never know.

CHAPTER 7

Oxygen

Floating on his back in the placid tropical waters, William Trubridge took a deep breath and then began nibbling frantically at the Bahamian sky. With each carp-like gulp, he sucked air into his mouth and then swallowed it, allowing him to squeeze an extra liter or so into his already inflated lungs, which have a measured capacity of 8.1 liters (the average person can inhale three to four liters). Finally, eyes closed, he rolled onto his front, dipped his head under the water, and plunged downward. His progress was studiously unhurried—a few languid pulls and frog kicks brought him thirty feet below the surface, where water pressure is twice as high as air pressure at the surface. As the pressure compressed the air in his lungs, his buoyancy decreased. By forty feet down, gravity had effectively reversed: he was now denser than water, free-falling deeper and deeper with no further effort. A one-pound weight around his neck kept his head pointed downward.

In a television studio back in New Zealand, where it was breakfast time, Trubridge's parents were watching uneasily. Two years earlier, in 2014, Trubridge had attempted to break his own record for the deepest unassisted freedive: no fins, no diving sleds, no breathing aids. TVNZ had broadcast the attempt live as Trubridge plunged to a depth of 102 meters (335 feet), grabbed a tag that had been Velcroed to the depth marker, and then reascended. He hadn't quite made it, blacking out after being hauled the last thirty feet to the surface by his safety divers. A similar blackout forty feet below the surface in 2006 had stopped his breathing for more than 20 seconds and, by some accounts, permanently robbed him of his sense of taste (a loss he now attributes to a "dodgy nasal spray"). Now he was trying the same 102-meter dive, plummeting downward in the sheltered waters of a saltwater cavern off the shores of the Bahamas' Long Island, again on live TV.

When Trubridge was eighteen months old, his parents had sold their house in northern England and bought a sailboat to carry the family on a long odyssey across the Atlantic, through the Caribbean, and eventually across the Pacific to New Zealand. "So I was brought up on the boat," he later recalled. "I was always around in the water, playing, snorkeling." Now, at thirty-six, Trubridge was the most decorated living freediver in the world, having set seventeen world records in the sport's various disciplines. (In this sport more than any other except BASE jumping, the qualifier "living" matters: Russian diver Natalia Molchanova, whose forty-one world records dwarfed Trubridge's paltry total, disappeared off the coast of Spain while giving a freediving lesson in 2015.) As he approached his target depth, his diving watch beeped to alert him; eyes still closed, he reached out a groping hand, grabbed the tag, and began kicking upward. Now, with his lungs compressed to the size of fists, the hard part began, a struggle against the downward pull of gravity. Halfway up, he felt his consciousness fading as the lack of oxygen asserted itself. Back in Auckland, his mother, too, looked like she was about to pass out as she struggled to answer the morning host's vapid questions.

Trubridge refocused and kept kicking. Finally, after 4 minutes and 14 seconds under the surface, he burst to the surface, gasping deep gulps of air and fumbling to remove his noseclip. "I'm okay," he mumbled, flashing the required hand signal to indicate he was under control. Seconds passed in agonizing suspense until, finally, the judges held up white cards to indicate a fair dive and the crowd—both in the Bahamas and in the Auckland studio—erupted in cheers.

There is no limit more fundamental—to endurance, and to life itself—than oxygen. We grasp its importance viscerally, in the lung-bursting gasps of physical exhaustion and the mounting panic of breath-holding. But does lack of oxygen actually stop us? The exploits of freedivers like William Trubridge and of mountaineers who ascend to the highest places on earth, where the air contains a third as much oxygen as at sea level, suggest that asphyxia's bark may be worse than its bite. By studying these extreme adventurers, scientists are learning to differentiate between when the body wants more oxygen and when it *needs* it, and their findings are reshaping our understanding of the role oxygen plays in the limits of endurance back at sea level. The urge to breathe (which is actually driven by a build-up of carbon dioxide rather than a lack of oxygen) turns out to be a warning signal that you can choose to ignore—up to a point.

For centuries, European travelers returned from voyages across the globe with improbable tales of pearl divers in the Caribbean, Asia, and the South Pacific who could dive down more than 100 feet, staying submerged for three or four (or, in some of the less plausible accounts, up to fifteen) minutes. But these traditional diving cultures had largely disappeared by the twentieth century, victims of new fishing and pearl-growing techniques. By 1949, when an Italian air force pilot named Raimondo Bucher wagered 50,000 lire that he could dive to nearly 100 feet on a single breath, most scientists thought such a feat would be fatal. After all, the volume of a gas is inversely proportional to its pressure—so at a depth of 100 feet, where pressure is quadrupled, your lungs will collapse to a quarter their normal size.

But Bucher made it, successfully grabbing a baton from a scuba diver waiting on the ocean floor off the island of Capri, and kicking off the modern era of competitive freediving—a sport whose focus on ever-greater depths remains controversial among those who see freediving as a means of exploring the ocean on its own terms rather than a form of underwater Russian roulette. These days there are a confusing array of freediving disciplines depending on the aids allowed, like fins and descending weights. In the "no limits" discipline, which permits weighted sleds for descending and self-inflating balloons to speed the ascent, Austrian daredevil Herbert Nitsch holds the record of just over

700 feet, set in 2007. He tried for 800 feet in 2012 but blacked out on the way to the surface and suffered the equivalent of several strokes, with lasting neurological consequences that affected his ability to walk and talk. (On his website, Nitsch claims this failed dive as a world record; the international freediving association doesn't recognize records unless the diver successfully completes a safety protocol after surfacing.)

Trubridge's record dive of 335 feet, with no aids other than the one-pound weight around his neck, is the one that's easiest to comprehend. But there's an even simpler category recognized by the freediving association: static apnea, which involves simply holding your breath for as long as possible. Floating facedown in a swimming pool with a spotter beside you avoids freediving complications like water pressure and decompression illness, conserves the oxygen needed to swim down and up, and allows you to push right to your limits without having to guess whether you'll have enough oxygen left to return to the surface. This last point is both a blessing and a curse—like the difference between Shackleton's out-and-back South Pole expeditions and Henry Worsley's one-way treks. Knowing that he could stop at any point, without needing to retrace his steps, is what allowed Worsley to push himself so fatally far. The current record holder in static apnea is a Frenchman named Stéphane Mifsud, who on a Monday afternoon in 2009 managed to stay submerged in his local pool for a hard-to-fathom 11 minutes and 35 seconds.

(Despite the discipline's apparent simplicity, the status of the record isn't without controversy. A Serbian diver named Branko Petrović now holds the Guinness record at 11:54, but he failed to adhere to the international freediving association's rules about announcing the attempt and not receiving assistance at the end of the breath-hold. Mifsud himself was accused on diving message boards of cheating, perhaps by inhaling oxygen through the vents in the swimming pool prior to his record performance—a charge unsupported by any evidence. The record for breath-holding after inhaling pure oxygen, a feat made famous by magician David Blaine's 17-minute hold in 2008, now stands at 24:03, by Spanish freediver Aleix Segura. But even Segura, after his performance, conceded that oxygen-assisted breath-holds were merely "a spectacle and experimental field rather than true apnea/freediving as a sport, which is what we all care about.")

Mifsud trains like an endurance athlete, putting in months of running, cycling, and swimming, including grueling Ironman triathlons. Only after his aerobic fitness is sharpened does he move to what he calls the "apprentice fish" stage, adding 30-second breath-holds to his cycling, repeated 20 times with a 15-second break between each one. Eventually, he moves into the water, spending as much as two hours, out of a six-hour training day, without breathing. His lung capacity is a remarkable 11 liters. But he and Trubridge and pretty much everyone else agree that, at the sharp end of the competition in any freediving discipline, the barriers are primarily mental, not physical. By the time he's been underwater for nine or ten minutes, the pain is like lying on a searing barbecue grill. His heart is beating every three seconds, and—worryingly—the urge to breathe has nearly disappeared. "You have to find the mental strength to continue," he says. "I tell myself that if I feel pain, it means I'm still alive."

There's a reason Mifsud's record was set in a swimming pool, and it's not just to ensure that he didn't cheat. Something close to magic occurs when you submerge your face in water—a vestigial reflex that we share with all mammals, both terrestrial and aquatic. In 1894, Nobel Prize–winning physiologist Charles Richet began publishing the results of a series of gruesome experiments in which he tied off the windpipes of ducks and timed how long they took to die. Some were strangled in open air, and lived for an average of 7 minutes; others were dunked underwater and survived for an average of 23 minutes. Richet (who, in addition to winning a Nobel Prize for work on anaphylactic reactions, was a dedicated researcher of the paranormal, coining the term *ectoplasm* nearly a century before the movie *Ghostbusters*) concluded that immersion in water had triggered a set of automatic responses, including a dramatic slowing of the heartbeat, that conserved oxygen.

These responses are now collectively known as the "mammalian dive reflex," or in the more poetic formulation of Swedish-American researcher Per Scholander, the "Master Switch of Life." When a Weddell seal dives, its heart rate immediately drops to a tenth of its usual value, helping it stay underwater for more than forty-five minutes. Scholander found a similar, though less extreme, response in human volunteers—even when he had them perform a vigorous workout while lying on the bottom of a water-filled wooden tank holding lead weights, which would normally make their heart rate shoot up. Trubridge's pulse drops into the 20s during his record dives; other freedivers have recorded values in the teens, below the minimum that physiologists once assumed were needed to maintain consciousness.

Another key part of the dive reflex is massive peripheral vasoconstriction: the blood vessels in your arms and legs squeeze nearly shut, sending blood flooding back to your core, where it maintains the crucial oxygen supply to your heart and brain for as long as possible. This shift of blood volume to your torso also helps your lungs resist collapse under the pressure of deep dives, since fluids (unlike air) are nearly incompressible. All it takes to trigger these changes is dunking your face in cool water; in fact, the sensors appear to be primarily around the nose, lending credence to the idea that splashing cold water on your face really can calm you down.

There are also more subtle responses, like the "spleen vent." The spleen mainly acts as a blood filter, but it also holds a reservoir of oxygen-rich red blood cells that can be deployed in emergencies. In seals, the organ is basically a natural scuba tank: it can hold more than twenty liters of red blood cells, and during dives it contracts like a wrung-out sponge, shrinking by 85 percent as it pushes the blood into circulation. Humans aren't quite so splenically gifted, but they do benefit from an infusion of oxygen-rich blood from the spleen, not only during dives but during any prolonged exercise to exhaustion. In one study, members of the Croatian national freediving team were compared to untrained subjects, some of whom had (for reasons unrelated to the study) had their spleens removed. They completed a series of five maximal breath-holds with their faces immersed in cold water to stimulate the dive reflex, separated by two minutes of recovery. In the subjects with spleens, both trained and untrained, their times progressively improved after the first attempt thanks to the infusion of extra blood, with benefits that lasted for more than an hour. In the spleenless subjects, the times remained unchanged throughout the five attempts.

For experienced freedivers, monitoring these subtle bodily responses provides a crucial gauge of how a dive is going. Hanli Prinsloo, a South African freediving coach, divides the progress of a dive into four stages. First is a subtle "awareness phase," where the urge to breathe begins to assert itself in your consciousness. If you push past that, you'll start to feel involuntary contractions in your diaphragm—a response to the buildup of carbon dioxide in your blood rather than the lack of oxygen. This you can safely (but temporarily) ignore, if you're willing to suffer. Then comes the welcome rush of fresh blood from the spleen, offering a psychological boost and allowing you to extend your dive. Finally, when your oxygen-hungry brain senses that its supply really is threatened, you black out, entering the neural equivalent of standby mode to conserve energy. You have to sense the progress of the first three stages to make sure stage four doesn't happen underwater (or better yet, Prinsloo says, at all). If it does, your larynx will reflexively close to keep water out of your lungs. But if someone doesn't get you to the surface within a matter of minutes, you'll eventually take one last big gasp, searching for oxygen, and drown.

The fact that people can dive to three hundred feet or hold their breath for nearly twelve minutes tells us that oxygen's absolute limits aren't quite as constrictive as they feel—that we're protected by layer upon layer of reflexive safety mechanisms. And there's a curious footnote to this process. Diving reflexes are controlled by the autonomic nervous system, which quarterbacks a wide range of bodily functions like heart rate, breathing, and digestion that are mostly outside of our conscious control. But if you strap a heart-rate monitor onto a seal, you find that its heart rate begins to plummet just *before* it dives into the water. The same is true in humans, though our responses are less pronounced and much more variable. In fact, once you've ingrained the behavior with a few practice trials, your heart rate will begin to drop as soon as you're instructed to dunk your head—even if the order is then countermanded and you stay dry. Tim Noakes would call this "anticipatory regulation": your brain uses knowledge that is gathered consciously, like an impending dive or a looming finish line, to activate or deactivate safety mechanisms that are otherwise purely unconscious.

That doesn't mean the brain always gets it right. The Divers Alert Network, which tracks accidents in both scuba and breath-hold diving around the world, reported 57 fatal freediving accidents in 2014. That's more than the 20 to 30 cases per year reported a decade ago, but down from the high of more than 70 in 2012. And even those who make it back to the surface alive sometimes pay a lasting price: William Trubridge's lost sense of taste; Herbert Nitsch's stroke-induced difficulties walking and talking. The reason we have such elaborate defense mechanisms against running out of oxygen is that the consequences are so dire.

Freedivers offer a graphic illustration of how the human body copes when its oxygen supply is completely shut off. But to understand how we cope with varying degrees of oxygen scarcity, it's useful to consider the opposite topographical extreme. If you climb out of the ocean in Monterey, stash your snorkel and flippers, and start walking inland, the air around you will get progressively thinner. That's because you're ascending through a massive ocean of air—the atmosphere—so the higher you go, the less of that weight is pressing down on you from above. When you reach the town of Mariposa, in the Sierra Nevada foothills at 1,949 feet above sea level, the amount of oxygen in each breath will have dropped by a mostly imperceptible 6 percent. Up the road in Mammoth Lakes, at 7,880 feet, it's down 24 percent—and you'll notice it. And by the time you scramble up the nearby summit of Mount Whitney, 14,504 feet up and with 41 percent less oxygen than normal, there's a good chance you'll have a splitting headache.

One of the first descriptions of altitude illness comes from a Chinese history written around 30 B.C.E. It describes a voyage between China and modern-day Afghanistan via the "Great Headache Mountain" and its lesser cousin, the "Little Headache Mountain," during which the travelers (and their asses and cattle) suffered from headaches and vomiting—classic signs of acute mountain sickness. Still, it wasn't until 1648, when French polymath Blaise Pascal deputed his brother-in-law to carry a mercury-filled barometer from the lowest point in the city of Clermont to the top of a nearby hill, that the crucial link between elevation and thinner air became clear. Over the next few centuries, scientists gradually pieced together the role of oxygen in respiration and the consequences of not getting enough. One notable early milestone, three centuries before athletes began sleeping in altitude tents: Robert Hooke tested the world's first artificial altitude chamber in 1671, sealing himself with cement into an airtight wooden cask that was submerged underwater in another cask, then using bellows and valves to expel air from the inner cask until his ears began to pop.

The invention of hot-air balloons offered a simpler (though no less dangerous) way of studying the effects of altitude. Within a few years of the first manned flight in 1783, physiologists and adventurers were ascending to extreme heights and reporting curious reactions to thin air: racing hearts, labored breathing, dizziness, and sometimes even numbness and paralysis. In 1799, a balloonist mounted on a horse (for reasons that history does not record) ascended until the horse started bleeding from its nose and ears. One key observation was that experienced balloonists seemed less likely to suffer from these problems, suggesting that repeated exposure to thin air triggered some form of adaptation. By the time the French balloon Zenith was launched in 1875, its passengers knew enough to bring supplemental oxygen to breathe. Still, all three men on board passed out as they exceeded 26,000 feet. Two hours later, one of them woke up as the balloon plummeted back to earth, and found that his companions, their eyes half-shut and their mouths open and full of blood, had died. Death by balloon was by no means uncommon at the time, thanks to fires, crash landings, and other mishaps—but the Zenith incident showed that at high enough altitudes, the air itself could be lethal.

Meanwhile, mountaineers were climbing ever-higher peaks—Mont Blanc, at nearly 16,000 feet, in 1786; Chimborazo, a 21,000-foot strato-volcano in Ecuador that was believed for a time to be the highest point on earth, in 1880—and encountering similar problems. (Chimbo-razo does still hold the distinction of being the farthest point from the earth's center, since the planet is thicker near the equator.) It was during a failed expedition to Chimborazo in 1802 that German naturalist Alexander von Humboldt first drew the link between lack of oxygen and the debilitating symptoms of altitude illness.

The highest peak of all, we now know, is Mount Everest, at 8,848 meters (29,029 feet). By the early 1920s, when the first British expeditions to the mountain began, climbers understood that gradual exposure to higher elevations could limit altitude illness. And unlike rapid balloon ascents, it was almost impossible *not* to acclimatize to some degree, given the arduous and unmapped five-week trek needed to reach the foot of the mountain. But even with that knowledge, it was still unclear whether the ascent was physically possible. The summit of Everest, scientists had determined, would offer barely a third as much oxygen as at sea level. Could men and women remain conscious under such conditions, let alone exert enough muscular force to climb through treacherous ice and snow?

In 1924, on the third British expedition in four years, soldier-turned-mountaineer Edward Norton made it to 28,126 feet—less than a thousand feet from Everest's summit. He turned back because, in addition to extreme breathlessness, he was seeing double by this point and as a result having great difficulty figuring out where to step in the treacherous terrain. Two days later, Norton's expedition-mates George Mallory and Andrew Irvine made another summit push, this time hauling clunky portable oxygen tanks on their backs to fight the altitude. Mallory was the man who, when asked by a *New York Times* reporter why he was returning to Everest for a third time, had famously replied "Because it's there." To this day, no one is sure whether or not Mallory and Irvine made it to the summit; either way, they never returned. They weren't the first to die on Everest: two local porters had already perished on that expedition, one from a cerebral hemorrhage triggered by the altitude; seven porters had died in an avalanche on the previous British expedition two years earlier. And they wouldn't be the last.

"No one cares for the prospect that they might become a cabbage." This was the fear lurking in the thin air on a clear May evening in 1978 as Reinhold Messner dictated notes into his miniature tape recorder at 26,000 feet above sea level. He and his climbing partner, Peter Habeler, were crammed into an ice-encrusted tent on Everest's South Col, preparing for an assault on the summit the next morning. Piles of snow surrounded them inside the tent, waiting to be melted over the weakly burning flame of their cooker; their sleeping bags were frozen rigid. The conversation rambled.

"Well, I'll tell you this much," Habeler said. "I'm turning back before I start going out of my mind."

"Me, too!"

"If I notice any symptoms that could mean brain damage, I'm calling a halt."

"If our speech gets affected or we notice any disturbance of balance or anything like that, then we must certainly turn back," Messner agreed.

From a geographical perspective, they weren't venturing into the unknown. A total of sixty men and two women had already reached the summit of Everest by this time, following in the footsteps of Edmund Hillary and Tenzing Norgay's first ascent in 1953. But all of them had used supplemental oxygen—an aid that Messner felt diminished both the accomplishment and the experience. "Even the highest mountains begin to shrink if they are besieged by hundreds of porters, attacked with pegs and oxygen apparatus," he argued. "In reaching for an oxygen cylinder, a climber degrades Everest to the level of a six-thousand-meter peak." He and Habeler had decided, instead, to make their attempt without extra oxygen—to see just how far humans could make it under their own power. "I want to climb until I either reach the top of the mountain," Messner wrote, "or I can go no further."

The two men had good reason to be apprehensive about their chances. After more than half a century, no one had yet managed to exceed the height reached by Edward Norton in 1924 without oxygen. Physiologists had debated what it would take to bridge that last 1,000 feet, and their conclusions weren't encouraging. In 1929, the eminent Italian scientist Rodolfo Margaria put himself and three unfortunate students through a grueling series of experiments that involved cycling in an altitude chamber at progressively decreasing pressures. Plotting a line through the data, he found they would be incapable of any further work once the pressure dropped to 300 millimeters of mercury. Since the estimated pressure at Everest's peak was 240 mmHg, he concluded that reaching it without oxygen would be impossible. A decade later, a similar analysis by Yandell Henderson at Yale, based on field measurements of acclimatized climbers from scientific expeditions to peaks around the world, reached the same conclusions: near the summit, Henderson wrote, "the rate of ascent must approach zero: in other words, a minimum of progress in an unlimited amount of time."

Messner, a bearded and ornery Italian from the German-speaking province of South Tyrol, was already a controversial figure in climbing circles. In his first Himalayan expedition, he and his brother Günther blazed a new route to the summit of Nanga Parbat, the ninth-highest mountain (and among the deadliest) in the world. But Günther, suffering from altitude illness, was killed in an ice avalanche on the way down, and other members of the expedition subsequently accused Messner (who himself lost seven toes to frostbite) of putting his thirst for glory ahead of his brother's safety—a charge he strongly denied. Messner was an early advocate of "alpine style" climbing, emphasizing rapid and lightly equipped ascents by small, self-sufficient teams rather than the "siege tactics" favored by big expeditions at the time. In 1975, he and Habeler completed the first alpine-style ascent of an 8,000-meter peak (just over 26,000 feet), scaling Gasherbrum I without oxygen in just three days.

The next big goal was clear, and Messner and Habeler settled on a motto: "Everest by fair means"—or not at all. The publicity surrounding the attempt (another talent of Messner's that irked fellow climbers) stirred up plenty of controversy. Experts, the *New York Times* reported, were "almost unanimous in declaring an ascent without oxygen to be certain suicide." But not everyone was so skeptical. A few days before his flight to Nepal, Messner received a letter from Edward Norton's son: "My father certainly believed," it read, "that, given the right conditions, Everest could be climbed without oxygen."

That caveat—"given the right conditions"—was a crucial one. As all Himalayan climbers soon learn, weather and snow conditions are as important to success as fitness and acclimatization. In their first summit push, Habeler developed food poisoning at Camp III and had to descend; Messner pushed on with two Sherpas, but the three men were then caught by a violent storm at the South Col and trapped in their tent for two full days in tent-shredding winds of up to 125 miles per hour and temperatures that plunged to −40 degrees Fahrenheit. By the time Messner and Habeler returned to the South Col for their final attempt, more than two weeks later, even they had begun to doubt whether their goal was attainable.

Sure enough, the morning of May 8 dawned windy and overcast. A squall of sleet slapped the two men in the face when they finally exited their tent, after the breath-sapping two-hour ordeal of getting dressed. They decided to push on anyway, the deepening snow eventually forcing them to scramble up challenging but snow-free rock ridges instead. To save breath, they communicated in sign language, scratching messages—an arrow pointing up or down—in the snow with their ice axes. By the time they reached the final approach, eight hours later, they were barely crawling forward, collapsing into the snow to rest every ten to fifteen steps. Finally, shaking with emotion and tears running down their cheeks as they gasped for air, they lay at the summit. Messner's description of the moment: "I am nothing more than a single, narrow, gasping lung, floating over the mists and the summits."

The successful climb caused physiologists to reassess the theoretical feasibility of a feat that was, after all, now clearly feasible in practice. A major research expedition to Everest three years later measured physiological responses all the way to the summit; another study had eight volunteers spend forty days in an altitude chamber simulating a full Everest ascent while being poked, prodded, and driven to exhaustion. The revised numbers suggested, not surprisingly, that Messner and Habeler's oxygen-free ascent was indeed possible—but just barely. Others soon repeated the feat (as of June 2016, there had been 197 oxygen-free summits out of a total of 7,646 by 4,469 people, according to the Himalayan Database), including Messner himself, who returned for a successful solo attempt from the Tibet side in 1980.

To physiologists, though, it remained an intriguing coincidence that the capacity of humans to survive in thin air should just happen to reach its absolute limit at the highest point on the planet. "If some evolutionary biologist can think of a reason for this," veteran high-altitude physiologist John West wrote in the *Annals of the New York Academy of Sciences* in 2000, "it would be very interesting to know about it." Coincidences, of course, do happen. But given all that we've learned about how finish lines and other endpoints influence the body's safety circuitry, I can't help but suspect that, if tectonic forces had given us a 30,000-foot peak instead of Everest's 29,029, someone would eventually scale it without supplementary oxygen.

In January 2013—midsummer in Australia, where my wife and I were living at the time—I started training for my first marathon. I'd been running seriously for more than twenty years, give or take a few interruptions, so I had a pretty good idea of how I would respond to the regimen. I had a good training group, a great coach, and the extra motivation of knowing I would be writing up my experiences for *Runner's World*, since I was also testing Samuele Marcora's brain endurance training protocol (which I'll describe in Chapter 11). I had been ill the previous fall and lost a lot of fitness, so in March I decided to check my progress by entering a low-key half-marathon. My time of 1:15:08 wasn't terrible, but it was a bit disappointing. At thirty-seven, I was no longer in my prime, but only a few years earlier I had been able to run similar times in training as medium-hard tempo runs. Clearly I still had work to do to get ready for the big day.

A month later, stronger and fitter, I entered another half-marathon as a final tune-up. This one went swimmingly: I felt good, paced myself well, and finished knowing I'd pushed as hard as I could. My time was better—1:12:55—but not by much. This time I had more difficulty coming up with excuses. I had put in three months of consistent mileage and hard-but-not-overzealous workouts, without any significant injuries or setbacks. If you had asked for an over-under before the race, I would have said 1:10:00. I was bummed, but eventually (this is the advantage of being a running science geek) I came up with a plausible alibi: altitude.

I was living in Canberra at the time, which is an inland city at the very modest elevation of just over 1,900 feet. Typically people don't start thinking about the effects of thin air until they're over 3,000 feet—in fact, in some studies of altitude training, the *low*-altitude control group lives at over 3,000 feet. But shortly after my disappointing half-marathon, I was interviewing some scientists at the Australian Institute of Sport (AIS), which is based in Canberra. A physiologist named Laura Garvican told me a story about when the AIS was first built and they were calibrating all the sophisticated testing equipment in the labs. Despite their best efforts, the VO_2max values they measured kept turning out slightly lower than the same athletes had recorded at other labs. Eventually they began to wonder whether the altitude might be having an effect after all—so they decided to test it using a pressurized chamber to vary the effective altitude.

The study, which was published in 1996, found a curious pattern.

In untrained subjects, there was no difference between sea level and Canberra. But in trained cyclists, VO_2max dropped by an average of 6.8 percent at 1,900 feet, and the effect seemed to be caused by a decline in the amount of oxygen ferried by the blood to the working muscles. Endurance athletes have hearts that pump so powerfully that their blood barely has time to load up with oxygen as it rushes past the lungs. Even at sea level, about 70 percent of male endurance athletes start to see measurable drops in arterial oxygen levels during all-out exercise, when the heart is pumping most powerfully. (The pattern is even more pronounced in women and older athletes.) Add in the slightly lower ambient oxygen levels at mild altitude like Canberra, and blood oxygen levels decline enough to affect how much oxygen your muscles are getting.

That same pattern, it turns out, is found among the best runners in the world, and even among those who grew up at much higher altitudes. When researchers from the University of British Columbia traveled to the highlands of Kenya to assess the lung and oxygen-processing capacity of the country's peerless distance runners, they found a similar prevalence of "exercise-induced arterial hypoxemia"— reduced levels of oxygen in the blood during heavy exercise—as in other populations. "These are the most fit people in the world," UBC researcher Bill Sheel told me, "but their blood gas looks like someone who might present at an ICU."

I could comfortably assume, then, that my VO_2max was probably a bit lower because of the altitude—but it wasn't immediately obvious why that should make me race slower at distances like a half-marathon. After all, a good distance runner might sustain an average of 85 percent of her VO_2max over the course of 13.1 miles; a marathoner might average 80 percent. Outside the lab, we seldom operate right at the limits of VO_2max, because the effort is too great to sustain for longer than about 10 minutes. At no point in my half-marathons was I *directly* limited by an inability to deliver more oxygen to my muscles. The same is true for long-distance races, and training studies have found that increases in VO_2max aren't necessarily proportional to increases in race performance. So why does VO_2max matter—if it does at all?

A. V. Hill and his successors were not wrong. VO_2max really is a pretty good predictor of performance. It can't pick the winner from a group of well-matched athletes (or well-matched couch potatoes, for that matter). But in a diverse group of people, you can reliably assume that those with higher VO_2max will outperform those with lower values in tests of endurance, even at long distances like a half-marathon where no one actually reaches their VO_2max. It's no coincidence that Norwegian cross-country skier Bjørn Dæhlie, who for many years held the unofficial mantle of the highest measured VO_2max in the world, was also at one point the most decorated Winter Olympic athlete in history, with twelve medals, eight of them gold. He was reportedly able to process and use 96 milliliters of oxygen per kilogram of body weight each minute; a typical healthy adult might manage 40.

It's worth taking the exact test numbers with a grain of salt. When I asked Stephen Seiler, a prominent American-born sports scientist who has worked in Norway since 1997, about Dæhlie's famous test, he was skeptical. He had seen the data but suspected there might have been a calibration problem. In the 1990s, when Dæhlie notched the value, Norway was locked in a fiercely competitive cross-country skiing "cold war" with Sweden, Russia, Italy, and other countries. "I think they knew it was a bad test at the time," Seiler says, "but let the media get wind of it to scare the competition." In 2017, Seiler and several other Norwegian sports scientists published a manuscript called "New Records in Human Power," echoing the title of a famous 1937 study from the Harvard Fatigue Lab, in which they pegged the highest reliably reported VO_2max values at around 90 ml/kg/min, seen in cyclists and cross-country skiers. Corresponding values in women are about 15 percent lower, thanks to higher levels of body fat and lower levels of oxygen-carrying hemoglobin in their blood; the highest reported value was about 78 ml/kg/min, again in a cross-country skier.

(A telling postscript: whether or not the number was accurate, Dæhlie lost the unofficial VO_2max record in the fall of 2012 to another Norwegian, an eighteen-year-old cyclist named Oskar Svendsen, who according to Norwegian media reports notched a lab score of 97.5 ml/kg/min and went on to win the junior time trial at the world cycling championships a few weeks later. After a few much-hyped but rocky years as a young pro, Svendsen retired in 2014, at age twenty. VO_2max is important, but it's not destiny.)

Still, the overall picture is that subtle differences in oxygen availability do affect performance. A later study by AIS scientists confirmed that Canberra's altitude didn't just lower VO_2max; it also slowed race times. Conversely, as we saw in Chapter 2, breathing pure oxygen seems to enhance endurance performance, even in situations (like a swim across the English Channel) where acute oxygen shortage isn't an issue. That why Yannis Pitsiladis, the scientist in charge of one of the projects aiming to beat Nike to a sub-two-hour marathon, flew to Israel at one point to scout the possibility of holding a marathon alongside the Dead Sea, near the lowest point on earth. At a quarter mile *below* sea level, the air there has about 5 percent more oxygen than at sea level, offering a potential (though, for now, hypothetical) boost. One of the key researchers on the performance-enhancing effects of oxygen? A guy named Roger Bannister, who published "The Effects on the Respiration and Performance During Exercise of Adding Oxygen to the Inspired Air" in the *Journal of Physiology* just over two months after breaking the four-minute-mile barrier in 1954. Boosting the air's oxygen content from the standard 21 percent to 66 percent, he found, allowed him to double his time to exhaustion on a steep uphill treadmill test.

One intriguing explanation for the limiting role of oxygen comes from research on "cerebral oxygenation"—the life-sustaining flow of blood to the brain. When you start exercising, the brain's oxygen levels initially rise, feeding the increased neuronal activity involved in sending instructions to muscles and monitoring effort. Then levels settle into a steady plateau—until you approach your limits. As you breathe more and more heavily, the carbon dioxide levels in your blood fall, which in turn makes the blood vessels leading to your brain constrict. (The same thing happens when you deliberately hyperventilate, causing you to get dizzy and eventually black out.) The resulting shortage of oxygen in the brain might directly interfere with muscle recruitment, or it might contribute to the sensation of fatigue signaling you to slow down or stop.

In 2010, researchers at the University of Lethbridge, in Canada, showed that the amount of oxygen in the brains of decent college-level competitive runners did indeed drop at the end of a 5K running trial. Then, four years later, another research team (including one of the same authors) ran a similar study on fifteen elite Kenyan runners. These subjects were truly world-class, with half-marathon bests of 62 minutes on average—and during their 5K trial, levels of oxygen in their brains stayed roughly constant right to the end. While it's hard to draw definitive conclusions from two small studies, the researchers suggested that being born at altitude and having very active childhoods ensured that the Kenyans were better equipped to maintain the brain's oxygen supply: they had more blood vessels to the brain, with thicker walls that were harder to squeeze shut.

An ingenious study by Guillaume Millet, whose work on muscle fatigue we discussed in the last chapter, offers further evidence that the endurance depends, at least in part, on oxygen levels in the brain. Millet had his subjects perform repeated arm flexes to exhaustion at simulated altitudes ranging from sea level to 23,000 feet, but he blocked off blood flow to and from the arm with a tight blood-pressure cuff. That meant that, despite the variations in altitude, the arm muscles received the same amount of oxygen (that is, none) in each case, producing the same degree of muscle fatigue and metabolite accumulation. Nonetheless, time to exhaustion was reduced by 10 to 15 percent at the highest altitude—a consequence, Millet concluded, of lower brain oxygenation.

There's one other line of evidence that points to a link between cerebral oxygenation and the limits of endurance. In 1935, an international team of scientists led by David Bruce Dill of the Harvard Fatigue Lab ventured to Chile, where they outfitted a mobile laboratory in a train car and journeyed from sea level to a sulfur mine on the upper slopes of a 20,000-foot-high volcano called Aucanquilcha, putting themselves and other volunteers through exhaustive experiments at various elevations along the route. In the process, they identified a puzzling and still-controversial phenomenon known as the "lactate paradox."

Under ordinary circumstances, you produce high levels of lactate in your muscles and blood when you "go anaerobic"—that is, when you're exercising so hard that your muscles can't get fuel quickly enough from the usual oxygen-dependent aerobic pathways. As you go to higher altitudes, with less oxygen in the air, you would expect to go anaerobic sooner, and produce more lactate at a given pace or power output. Instead, Dill's team observed the opposite: the higher they went, the lower the lactate levels they were able to produce at exhaustion. Extrapolating from their data (which has since been reproduced and reconfirmed many times) suggests that by the time you reach 23,000 feet, where oxygen levels are less than half their sea-level values, you won't be able to raise your lactate levels at all.

A series of studies by Markus Amann and his colleagues, involving 5K cycling time trials and rides to exhaustion at a range of simulated altitudes, offers a possible explanation for this seeming paradox. The higher the altitude, the weaker the brain's signals to the leg muscles, as measured by EMG electrodes, became. This reduced muscle activation was evident right from the start of each trial, before fatigue had a chance to set in, suggesting that the brain was throttling back muscular effort preemptively. And at the point of exhaustion, the muscles themselves showed *less* fatigue (as measured by electrical stimulation) at high altitudes than they did at sea level, despite the shortage of oxygen in the air. The debilitating exhaustion experienced by Reinhold Messner and other mountaineers, in other words, isn't because their muscles aren't getting enough oxygen; it's because their brains are in danger of running short—which, evolution has determined, is much more serious.

So is oxygen a "real" limiting factor in endurance? It seems convenient to make a distinction between ironclad limits imposed by your muscles and softer, more negotiable ones imposed by your mind. (As I mentioned earlier, my initial intention when I set out to write this book was to argue that the latter were far more common than the former.) The dichotomy works in some cases. While the world's best breath-holders certainly have some unique physiological skills and adaptations, it's clear that initial progress in breath-holding—going from one minute to three minutes, say—is mostly a matter of simply accepting and ignoring the rising sense of anguish and panic. It's in your head. At the same time, mountain climbers who don't adapt well to extreme elevation—and this seems to be largely genetic, unrelated to fitness or experience—often get sick and sometimes die at the elevations scaled by Messner. That's not in their heads.

But in practice, assigning the blame to mind or muscles is an often hopeless and sometimes misleading task. After all, the brain is part of the body. This was a point emphasized by Michio Ikai and Arthur Steinhaus in 1961, when they studied the psychological effects of surprise gunshots on muscle strength (see page 103): "[P]sychology," they wrote, "is a special case of brain physiology." In other words, feelings and emotions and urges are as physiologically real as changes in core temperature or decreases in hydration, and are mediated by chemical signals. So when oxygen levels in the brain drop, are we compelled by failing neurons or safety circuitry to slow down, or do we simply decide to slow down? Is there a difference? Whatever the answers (and I don't think we know them at this point), the outcome is clear. We slow down.

CHAPTER 8

Heat

Blame it on the Kentuckiana sun, which was beating down with its customary August fierceness. Or blame the untameable restlessness of boys who have just started a new school year, or the girls' soccer game getting under way on an adjacent field. For whatever reason, the football players on the practice field at Pleasure Ridge Park High School were not listening to their coach, Jason Stinson, as he called for his starters to take their positions for a scrimmage. Eventually, Stinson, who had taken over the head coaching job in the Louisville suburb that year after three years as an assistant, ran out of patience. "On the line," he roared. "If we're not going to practice, we're going to run!"

For the next thirty to forty minutes, the players ran "gassers," an all-too-familiar conditioning drill that involved sprinting back and forth across the field four times. A single gasser takes about a minute; after eight of them, some of the boys had slowed to a walk, enraging Stinson even more. He pulled eight of the worst offenders out of the line and had them start up-downs, a tougher drill that alternated between running on the spot and dropping to the ground, while the others continued running gassers. "We're gonna run," he told them, "until somebody quits!" During the twelfth gasser, a boy named David Englert, who had already quit the team three times only to return, walked off the field yet again. "Ding, ding, ding!" Stinson proclaimed. "We have a winner!"

Practice was over, and the players began to disperse. A sophomore named Max Gilpin was walking across the field to collect the equipment he had shed during the gassers, when his legs began to wobble.

Two of Gilpin's teammates propped him up and hauled him over to a nearby shade tree, where he lost consciousness. The teammates called for help; soon he was surrounded by assistant coaches, then loaded onto a Gator driven by the school's athletic director. He was doused in water and cooled with ice packs. Someone called 911. But it was too late: three days later, on August 23, 2008, at Kosair Children's Hospital, Max Gilpin died of complications stemming from heatstroke.

What's most chilling about Gilpin's death is how unsurprising it is. According to a tally kept by the National Center for Catastrophic Sport Injury Research, a total of 143 football players died from heatstroke between 1960 and 2016. The vast majority of those deaths were high schoolers, and they generally took place during summer practices, when the weather was hottest and the players were least fit. But even pros are not immune: the heatstroke death of Minnesota Vikings offensive tackle Korey Stringer, during a training camp in 2001, put the issue on front pages around the country, albeit briefly.

Gilpin's death was unique in one respect, though. Exactly a week after the fateful practice, Louisville's chief prosecutor announced that he had asked local police to open an investigation into the case—a first in heat-related sports deaths. Five months later, Jason Stinson was formally charged with reckless homicide, and another charge of wanton endangerment was subsequently tacked on. Gilpin had pushed beyond his physical limits—or rather, prosecutors argued, he had *been* pushed beyond his limits by Stinson's "barbaric practice," which according to some eyewitness accounts had involved denying water to the players.

Back in 1996, as Tim Noakes prepared for his famous keynote lecture at the American College of Sports Medicine, he had puzzled not over the fact that some people push themselves to death in the heat, but that most people don't. In some ways, Stinson's thirteen-day trial in 2009 became a tussle over this observation. The prosecution argued that Gilpin's death was a direct and foreseeable consequence of Stinson's actions; the defense countered that it was a tragic and unforeseeable aberration. Nearly a hundred players had been subject to Stinson's barbarism that afternoon; thousands more were doing similar drills across Kentucky, and more than a million boys around the country were suiting up for their high school football teams. The jury's task: to determine what, if anything, made Max Gilpin different.

In 1798, Sir Benjamin Thompson, a Massachusetts-born polymath who fled to Britain after the American Revolution, invented sous-vide cooking, and introduced the potato to Bavaria (where he was granted the title Count Rumford), sparked a revolution in the study of heat. The muscular exertions of two horses, he showed, could generate enough heat over the course of a few hours to boil 2.25 gallons of water. "It would be difficult to describe the surprise and astonishment expressed in the countenances of the bystanders," he reported, "on seeing so large a quantity of cold water heated and actually made to boil without any fire."

The human body, as Thompson's experiment suggested, is quite literally a furnace. It transforms the energy from food into mechanical work—and this transformation generates heat as a sometimes useful and sometimes inconvenient by-product. The harder you work, the more heat you generate. The first rigorous investigation of the efficiency of the human engine, which involved months of experiments on a professional cyclist named Melvin A. Mode in a Boston laboratory in 1911 and 1912, recorded typical values of 20 to 25 percent. For every 100 calories of food you eat, in others words, you might get 25 calories of useful work and 75 calories of heat. As wasteful as that sounds, it's surprisingly similar to the efficiency of a typical internal combustion engine.

The heat generated by your car's engine can be pretty useful on a cold day: it's what blasts through your heating vents to warm up the interior. The same is true for human heat production, which is why even extreme cold is rarely a limiting factor for endurance athletes, whose furnaces burn far hotter than most. "Under normal circumstances, it's very rare for people to reach the limits of their cold tolerance if they're appropriately dressed," says Ira Jacobs, a University of

Toronto researcher and former chief scientist with Canada's Department of National Defence.

For athletes, the biggest cold-related problems arise when your activity level changes, which happens if you get too tired to maintain the effort level that has been keeping you warm. And it's worse if your clothes get wet and lose their insulative powers. That's what happened during a notorious hiking competition on the moors of Yorkshire in 1964, when three young men died in above-freezing but rainy conditions—a tragedy investigated by Griffith Pugh, the physiologist who helped guide Edmund Hillary and Tenzing Norgay to the summit of Mount Everest. In the 1990s, Jacobs notes, the same type of "hiker's hypothermia" led to the deaths of four U.S. Rangers during training exercises in Florida, of all places. Once the furnace goes out, even mild cold can kill.

Far more common are the thermoregulatory problems that arise in hot weather, because the body is like a car with no air-conditioning: you've got no way of actively cooling yourself, so the best you can do is get rid of excess heat as quickly as possible. At rest, about 250 milliliters (half a pint) of blood per minute flows through the vessels near your skin, carrying heat away from your core and releasing it to the environment primarily through radiation (in the form of electromagnetic waves) and convection (as moving air carries it away). As a result, you're always giving off heat at a rate of about 100 watts, just like a lightbulb (except mostly at infrared rather than visible wavelengths), which perfectly balances the excess heat produced by the basal metabolic reactions that keep you alive.

Once you start pedaling your bike, that changes quickly. Because of the body's imperfect efficiency, cycling at 250 watts generates as much as 1,000 watts of excess heat. Running at 10 miles per hour produces a sizzling 1,500 watts. In response, the blood vessels in your skin dilate dramatically, allowing up to eight liters of blood per minute—a thirty-fold increase—to course through them and dump heat to the air around you. (The opposite happens in cold temperatures, leading to what scientists call "physiological amputation" as your body conserves heat by cutting off blood supply to extremities.) You also begin to sweat: the transformation of liquid water to vapor as sweat evaporates consumes energy, creating a powerful cooling effect on the skin. In very hot conditions, when the air temperature is comparable to or higher than your skin temperature, evaporation is the only effective cooling method you've got. And if it's so humid that sweat starts dripping off you instead of evaporating, the clock is ticking as your core temperature starts to inch upward.

At 3:45 P.M. on the day of Max Gilpin's death, Coach Stinson filled out and signed the daily weather records as his players took to the field. He noted a temperature of 94 degrees, with humidity, as measured by the school's hygrometer, of 32 percent. Plugging those two numbers into a chart produced a heat index of 94—one below the threshold of 95, at which rules about compulsory water breaks and removal of bulky equipment would kick in. It was hot, though not as hot as some of the previous practices that summer. When the heat index had soared to 103 a few weeks earlier, Stinson had run the practice with helmets off.

In that respect, Gilpin's death was unusual: it didn't happen on the first day, or even the first week, of summer practice. It was the team's sixth week, and every single one of their twenty-nine previous workouts had taken place with a heat index above 80, including five above 95. When you exercise repeatedly in hot conditions, your body's protective responses get progressively better: you sweat more heavily, starting at a lower temperature; your vessels dilate even wider to deliver heat-laden blood to the skin; and the total volume of blood in your body increases, allowing your heart rate to stay lower during exercise. This acclimatization process takes about two weeks, which is why organizations like the National Athletic Trainers' Association recommend limiting intensity and the use of full equipment during the first fourteen days of football practice each summer.

The idea that we can adapt to hot conditions has been known anecdotally for centuries. In 1789, for example, a British Army doctor in

India observed that heat-related health problems became less and less common after the first few days of each new military campaign. But it wasn't until the 1930s that the adaptation process was studied systematically. The impetus was a rash of heatstroke deaths—26 in 1926 alone—in South African gold mines as ever-deeper shafts, more than a thousand meters below the surface, penetrated into rocks that could be as hot as 140 degrees.

A young doctor named Aldo Dreosti was assigned by Rand Mines Ltd. to find a solution to this problem. The African workers in the company's City Deep mine in Johannesburg, where Dreosti was assigned, were already given an acclimatization period of up to fourteen days when they first started working underground, during which two workers would share a single shovel so that neither would work non-stop. But it clearly wasn't working, since twenty workers had died of heatstroke at City Deep between 1926 and 1931. And perhaps more important to the mine's owners, letting all workers undergo this acclimatization period when only a few seemed susceptible to heatstroke hurt the bottom line: "The financial position of the mine," Dreosti explained to colleagues at a mining symposium in 1935, "was such as to be profoundly affected by this loss of efficiency."

The challenge was to figure out which workers were most likely to be vulnerable to heat, and find the quickest way to prepare them for the rigors of underground work. To do this, Dreosti converted an unused hospital ward into a heat chamber crisscrossed with perforated pipes releasing steam, where up to fifty workers at time could undergo the "Heat Tolerance Test" he devised. The test involved stripping naked and shoveling piles of rock back and forth with a partner for one hour at a temperature of 95 degrees, overseen by a "specially trained native 'Boss Boy.'" After testing 20,000 workers in his chamber, Dreosti was able to divide his subjects into three groups based on how high and how quickly their body temperature rose, and assigned these groups either 4, 7, or 14-day acclimatization periods.

As shocking as some of Dreosti's work sounds to modern ears, it was strikingly successful in reducing heatstroke deaths at City Deep—

and in getting the miners working at full steam as quickly as possible. In the years that followed, researchers continued to tinker with the ideal acclimatization protocol. Studies during World War II, when Allied troops were preparing for combat in stifling jungle and desert environments, found that 60 to 90 minutes of moderate exercise per day in hot conditions would produce rapid physiological changes within a few days, with full acclimatization taking place within about two weeks. Simply living through a hot summer isn't enough; you have to stress your system with exercise. And that, as it turns out, is exactly what Max Gilpin and his teammates had been doing each day at practice for six weeks by the time he died. Whatever culpability Stinson had, in other words, it wasn't a result of jumping into full practices too quickly.

In the late 1990s, researchers at Denmark's storied August Krogh Institute at the University of Copenhagen carried out a simple experiment to test the effects of core temperature on the limits of endurance. Seven cyclists completed a series of rides to exhaustion in hot and humid conditions, pedaling until they were physically unable to sustain a minimum cadence of 50 strokes per minute at the goal pace. Before each ride, they spent 30 minutes soaking up to the neck in cool, neutral, or warm water, so that their starting core temperatures were roughly 97, 99, or 101 degrees Fahrenheit. As expected, the riders lasted longest when they were precooled, more than doubling their performance compared to the preheated condition. But despite the large differences between trials, the cyclists' core temperatures at exhaustion were strikingly consistent. In nearly every ride by every rider, the thermometer read between 104.0 and 104.5 degrees at the moment of failure. It was as if, in crossing that critical threshold, a temperature-sensitive circuit-breaker had been tripped.

Sports scientists were quick to appreciate the potential performance benefits implied by the study. The Australian Olympic team brought ice baths to the sun-drenched 2004 games in Athens, so that athletes could plunge in shortly before their events. In 2008, they adopted a simpler and more practical approach, shipping seven slushie machines to Beijing and deploying them at the venues for track, cycling, soccer, triathlon, and several other sports. Just as the transformation of liquid water to vapor cools your skin when you sweat, the "phase change energy" of ice melting to water in your stomach provides an extra cooling boost beyond what you would get from simply drinking a cold drink. Tests by Australian sports scientists showed that a crushed ice slurry sweetened to the same degree as a sports drink could lower core temperatures by one degree Fahrenheit and, in consequence, boost endurance in the heat.

One curious fact about the slushies was they didn't just lower the athletes' initial temperature; in some cases, they also allowed them to push to a slightly higher core temperature before reaching exhaustion. The difference was minor—about half a degree Fahrenheit—but intriguing nonetheless. By drinking the slushies, researchers speculated, the athletes might have also cooled their brains as the ice passed through their mouth and throat. Earlier studies with goats and dogs whose brains were cooled by irrigating cold water through their noses had suggested that brain temperature, rather than core temperature (which is typically measured rectally), is what determines your ultimate thermal limits. If a slushie cools your brain, then your brain lets you keep pedaling a little longer even as the rest of your body heats up beyond its usual limits.

A related possibility is that you have temperature sensors in your stomach itself, where the slushie melts. Until recently, such a possibility would have been dismissed as fanciful. But in 2014, Ollie Jay and his colleagues at the University of Ottawa's Thermal Ergonomics Laboratory showed that they could alter sweat rate in cyclists by delivering warmed or cooled fluid directly to their stomachs via a tube inserted through the nose. Jay, who has since moved to the University of Sydney, notes that this may help explain the long-standing tradition in some cultures of drinking a hot drink like tea during scorching summer afternoons. By triggering the temperature receptors in your stomach, the hot drink ramps up your sweating response without heating the rest of your body, which has the net effect of cooling you down.

So is it brain temperature or stomach temperature that matters most? It's probably a bit of both—along with temperature signals from other parts of the body, like the skin. There's a reason athletes don ice-filled vests and cooling sleeves and drape ice towels over their necks: these interventions don't alter your core temperature, but they do influence how hot you *feel*—and that, in turn, dictates how hard you're able to push. Further evidence that perception is reality: a British study in 2012 showed that cyclists in a heat chamber went 4 percent faster when the thermometer was rigged to display a falsely low temperature (79 instead of 89 degrees Fahrenheit).

This perception-centered view runs counter to the prevailing notion that heat slows you down through its direct physiological effects on your body. But the truth is that few of us ever encounter the critical temperature threshold that makes people keel over in laboratory heat chamber tests. Instead, we instinctively—and perhaps unwillingly—moderate our pace to stay below that threshold. As South African sports scientist Ross Tucker has shown, when you set out to run a 10K on a hot summer day, your pace is slower *right from the start,* long before your body has even begun to warm up. Heat doesn't act like a light switch that flicks your muscles off; in most real-world situations, as Tucker explained to me, it's a dimmer switch, controlled by the brain for your own protection.

That doesn't mean your body is irrelevant. Max Gilpin had been training hard between his freshman and sophomore years in high school, hitting the weight room with his father two or three times a week for an hour or more per session. His father told him about his own steroid use as a younger man, and warned him about the dangers of these illicit drugs. Instead, he suggested Max take creatine, a legal over-the-counter supplement that helps enhance muscle gains.

By the time Max started tenth grade, he had packed on about 27 pounds since the previous year, and at 6'2" he weighed 216 pounds. He wasn't the biggest guy on the football team, but he was a substantial presence—pretty much the opposite, in fact, of a typical elite marathon runner.

In 2013, researchers at France's National Sport Institute collected anthropomorphic data on the top 100 marathoners in the world for each year between 1990 and 2011. They noticed a surprising trend: marathon runners were shrinking at an alarming rate. In 1990, the average top-100 runner had clocked in at just over 5'8" and 131 pounds; by 2011, those numbers had dropped to under 5'7" and 124 pounds. The reason, the researchers suspected, was simple: the heavier you are, the more heat you generate while running around. Tall people also have more skin surface area, which allows them to shed more heat by sweating—but the extra weight swamps the effects of the extra skin, putting bigger and taller runners at a subtle disadvantage. As marathoning became a big-money sport in the 1990s and 2000s, marathoners' bodies became ever more specialized for staying cool. At the opposite end of the spectrum, football players' bodies are optimized for a more brutal contest—and in particular, linemen like Max Gilpin, giant locomotives of destruction, are the most vulnerable, accounting for 50 of the 58 heatstroke deaths among football players between 1980 and 2009.

With each passing sprint, Gilpin's temperature, and his perception of that temperature, edged upward. After six gassers, Stinson began dismissing the fastest runners; after eight, he had the remaining players remove their helmets and keep going; after ten, they pulled off their jerseys and shoulder pads. Gilpin was not a fast runner, so he had no hope of an early reprieve—but he kept pushing himself nonetheless. "He was, to borrow a word from his adoring mother, a pleaser," *Sports Illustrated*'s Thomas Lake later reported. His father, who sometimes refused to drive him home after practice if he didn't perform well, was watching from the sidelines. Could Gilpin's eagerness to please have spurred him to push beyond his limits?

According to the critical temperature studies, he should have been unable to continue once his core temperature hit 104 degrees. It turns out, though, that critical temperature isn't quite as immovable as the initial studies suggested. Stephen Cheung, an avid cyclocross racer and environmental physiologist at Brock University in Canada, first explored this topic during his doctoral studies. In a military-funded experiment, he showed that fit, well-trained athletes could push to a higher core temperature during a treadmill test than less fit subjects—evidence that the brain's temperature settings can indeed be altered.

Cheung's most recent work provides even more remarkable evidence of the brain's power. He and his colleagues put a group of eighteen trained cyclists through a battery of physical and cognitive tests at 95 degrees Fahrenheit. Then half the cyclists received two weeks of training in "motivational self-talk" specifically tailored to exercising in heat, which basically involved suppressing negative thoughts like "It's so hot in here" or "I'm boiling," and replacing them with motivational statements like "Keep pushing, you're doing well." The self-talk group improved their performance on one of the endurance tests from 8 minutes to 11 minutes—and in doing so, pushed their core temperatures at exhaustion more than half a degree higher. "We're now pretty sure it's not just a physical thing," Cheung says of the critical temperature concept. "There seems to be a strong mental-psychological component to it." The right frame of mind, in other words, allows you to push beyond your usual temperature limits: "Even if you're already fit, you can still improve your *perception* of heat and how you perform in it."

There's still a mystery, though. Self-talk enabled Cheung's cyclists to push their core temperature a mere half-degree higher before collapsing from exhaustion; Max Gilpin's temperature eventually reached an organ-melting 109.4 degrees, five full degrees above the usual limit. We've traditionally viewed heatstroke as the last stop on a continuum: first you feel warm, then you're uncomfortably hot, then you get heat exhaustion, and finally, if you don't stop, you develop heatstroke. But most people are physically incapable of pushing their temperature to anywhere near 109 degrees. To reach that extreme, something different must be going on.

In 2002, a pair of doctors from the sunny climes of Saudi Arabia and Texas published a joint paper in the *New England Journal of Medicine* proposing a revised definition of heatstroke. It's not just about body temperature, they argued; heatstroke involves a "systemic inflammatory response" that ultimately triggers a cascade of escalating symptoms that lead to multi-organ failure. The body's defenses against heat, as we learned earlier, involve shunting blood toward the skin, where it releases heat. The flip side of this response is that the gut and other internal organs are starved of blood and oxygen. Eventually, this allows toxins that are normally corralled in the gut to begin leaking into the bloodstream, where they trigger a system-wide inflammatory surge. Heatstroke isn't just about getting hot; it's about a surge of inflammation that disables the body's normal temperature defenses.

So why does the inflammatory response spiral out of control in a few people? There's a long list of factors that nudge your heatstroke risk upward, but researchers at the U.S. Army Research Institute of Environmental Medicine, in a 2010 review, singled out three in particular: heavy, poorly ventilated clothing; preexisting illness; and the use of certain drugs such as amphetamines. Gilpin's football equipment ticked the first box. He likely ticked the second one, too: his stepmother told doctors that he'd had a headache and felt unwell that morning, and several of his friends provided similar testimony. (The medical evidence was inconclusive: his blood tests showed signs of viral infection but couldn't distinguish whether it started before or after he was admitted to hospital.) And the toxicology test at the hospital confirmed the third risk factor, too: Gilpin was taking Adderall, an amphetamine-based drug, to treat attention deficit disorder.

Perhaps the most famous heatstroke casualty in sports is the British cyclist Tom Simpson, who died less than a mile from the summit of Mont Ventoux on a sizzling day during the 1967 Tour de France. Simpson's will to win and capacity for self-punishment were notorious, and when he began zigzagging back and forth across the road then tumbled to the ground, his response—according to a stirring but probably apocryphal story—was to cry "Put me back on my bike!" He managed to pedal another quarter mile or so before collapsing again, and was dead long before a police helicopter ferried him to a nearby hospital.

Like Gilpin, Simpson had been sick in the days prior to his final ride. His mechanic recalled hosing diarrhea off his bike after the stage a few days earlier, thanks to an unpleasant stomach bug whose effects still lingered. But what cycling history remembers about Simpson is the amphetamines: at the time of his collapse, he had three pill tubes in his jersey, two empty and one half-full, and the autopsy confirmed their presence in his blood. The standard accounting of his death is that the pills impaired his judgment, leaving him "so doped that he did not know he had reached the limit of his endurance," as Britain's *Daily Mail* put it a few weeks later.

The truth is a little more complicated. In the 1980s, a biochemist (and enthusiastic marathon runner) at the University of Oxford, Eric Newsholme, proposed that fatigue during endurance exercise might result in part from changes in the concentration of neurotransmitters in the brain. That hypothesis didn't pan out, but it led to string of studies testing the effects of various brain-altering drugs on endurance: Paxil, Prozac, Celexa, Effexor, Wellbutrin, Ritalin, and others. Under normal conditions, the drugs had minimal effects; but in hot conditions, drugs that increased concentrations of the neurotransmitter dopamine in the brain had a dramatic effect.

Even at rest, subjects taking dopamine reuptake inhibitors (which increase the brain's dopamine levels; amphetamines are in this class of drug) had higher core temperatures, suggesting that the drugs altered the perception and internal regulation of heat. Once the subjects started exercising in the heat, they were able to push farther and harder, causing their temperatures to rise beyond their usual critical threshold—even though they didn't *feel* hotter. "Their 'safety brake' didn't work," explains Romain Meeusen, a physiologist at Vrije Universiteit Brussel in Belgium who conducted some of the key experiments. "They became capable of pushing into the danger zone without negative feedback from their central nervous system." This, he adds, is likely what happened to Tom Simpson.

At Jason Stinson's trial, a series of medical experts—including one who had initially been approached by the prosecution—testified that Gilpin's Adderall use had likely contributed to his susceptibility to heatstroke. Of course, millions of people in the United States take Adderall regularly, and this hasn't fueled an epidemic of heatstroke (although one study by University of Georgia researchers estimated that heat-related football deaths tripled between 1994 and 2009, a period during which prescriptions of Adderall and related drugs more than doubled among teens). By any measure, Gilpin's death was a very-low-probability event, a lightning strike with no single obvious cause. But the accretion of subtle risk factors—the Adderall, the illness, and perhaps the creatine (which some scientists believe can contribute to heat illness)—made Gilpin just a little more of a lightning rod than usual that afternoon.

On this list of contributing factors, one item is conspicuously absent: dehydration. This was the root of the criminal case, based on reports that Stinson had denied his players water during the practice, and on the general assumption that most problems in the heat stem from not drinking enough. Under scrutiny, the eyewitness descriptions of the football practice (the most damning of which came from Stinson's brother's ex-girlfriend, who was watching the girls' soccer game on an adjacent field) turned out to be misleading. The full team had three scheduled water breaks during the practice, and individual players were drinking between drills.

There was, to be sure, plenty of yelling. Even Stinson's attorney told the judge, "I think you can almost take judicial notice that Jason Stinson was being a jerk that day." But the boys drank, and the blood and urine tests performed when Gilpin arrived at the hospital showed that he was not even moderately dehydrated. That fact, more than anything else, is what convinced the jury to acquit Stinson after less than ninety minutes of deliberation. Contrary to the intuition drummed into us by a generation of public health messages, drinking more would not have saved Max Gilpin. And that, it turns out, is not the only piece of conventional wisdom about hydration that is wrong.

CHAPTER 9

Thirst

Pablo Valencia and Jesus Rios left the waterhole a few hours before dawn on August 15, 1905, loading their horses with a week's worth of pinole and three gallons of water. They were on their way to stake a claim for a "lost mine" that Valencia had discovered a few months earlier, in the remotest reaches of the Sonoran desert near the Arizona-Mexico border. But as they rode deeper into the sandy barrens, their mouths parching in the oven-dried air, they realized that they had misjudged their water needs. Valencia told Rios to take the horses and backtrack thirty-five miles to the waterhole to refill their canteens, and they arranged to rendezvous twenty-four hours later on the far side of a sierra in the distance. Valencia continued on foot to the claim site, where he collected samples and posted the requisite notices; Rios fetched the water and headed back into the desert. But the rendezvous didn't happen. One or both of them must have gone to the wrong hill, and they each wandered aimlessly until Rios gave up and left his partner for dead.

The human body is about 50 to 70 percent water, and it needs pretty much all of it. You're constantly losing water, not just from sweat but also from urine and more subtle leaks like the moisture in your breath. And, under normal circumstances, you're constantly replacing it by eating and drinking. Your fluid balance fluctuates a bit throughout the day thanks to meal and activity patterns, but from one day to the next it's regulated with remarkable precision. A 150-pound person typically carries around about forty liters of water, and that total is fixed to within less than a liter (one exception is the fluctuations that occur throughout a woman's menstrual cycle, which can add and then subtract more than two liters of retained water). When you fail to replace lost fluids, you start craving a drink, and your kidneys begin reabsorbing fluid that would otherwise become urine. If that's not enough to restore your internal balance, fluid will start draining out of your cells and into your veins and arteries to maintain the necessary volume of blood pumping through your body. These adjustments will buy you some time, but eventually your blood will get so concentrated that your brain will start shrinking as fluid is sucked out by osmosis, tearing delicate cerebral veins and ultimately killing you. According to calculations by U.S. Army researchers in a wilderness medicine textbook, you might last, in theory, for about seven days without water under ideal indoor conditions before reaching this critical point. If you're lost in a hot desert and travel only by night, your expected survival plummets to twenty-three hours; if you also travel during the day, it's sixteen hours.

Valencia was a vigorously fit forty-year-old ex-sailor-turned-prospector, deep-chested and strong-limbed—"indeed," a contemporary described him, "one of the best-built Mexicans known to me." But the circumstances were stacked against him: daytime temperatures hovering around 100 degrees, nighttime lows in the 80s, cloudless skies, and scant humidity. By the evening of his second day in the desert, after failing to find Rios, he was completely out of water and was forced to begin gargling his own urine. Rather than heading straight back to the waterhole, he decided to head north toward an old wagon trail in the hopes of finding help sooner. Along the way, he killed a few spiders and flies, but his mouth was so dry that he struggled to swallow them. On his fourth day in the desert, he caught and ate a scorpion; he was now drinking his urine, which by this time was "mucho malo"—very bad. He was already beating the odds, since half the victims of desert thirst in the area died within thirty-six hours, and nearly all within three days. But he didn't quit. Fueled by the dream of knifing Rios, who he believed had betrayed him to keep the lost mine for himself, he walked, then staggered, then crawled on.

Eight days after Valencia and Rios had set out from the waterhole, a scientist named William J. McGee, who had been camped there for one hundred days taking weather measurements, was woken from a deep sleep by an anguished, guttural roar. Rushing a quarter mile down the trail, he found Valencia—stark naked and shrunken to a skeleton. "[H]is lips had disappeared as if amputated, leaving low edges of blackened tissue; his teeth and gums projected like those of a skinned animal, but the flesh was as black and dry as a hank of jerky; his nose was withered and shrunken to half its length; his eyes were set in a winkless stare, with surrounding skin so contracted as to expose the conjunctiva, itself as black as the gums." He could barely see or hear, and his tongue had all but disappeared. He had covered between 100 and 150 miles on foot, and had crawled for the last seven miles across a stony and cactus-dotted plain, leaving him covered in deep cuts and scratches that were too dry to bleed.

But he lived. McGee slowly nursed him back to health with judicious amounts of water, coffee, and "bird fricassee with rice and shredded bacon," and presented the remarkable case report at a medical conference in 1906. Whether this constitutes a record of some sort is hard to say. Older editions of the *Guinness Book of World Records* note the case of Andreas Mihavecz, an eighteen-year-old Austrian who was locked up in a small-town jail in 1979 after being a passenger in a minor car accident and then, the arresting officers later testified, "simply forgotten." It wasn't until eighteen days later that a horrific stench emanating from the basement reminded them of Mihavecz's presence. While he had lost nearly fifty pounds, he too lived—presumably, medical experts speculated, because the basement cell was so unpleasantly dank that he was able to lick drops of condensation from the walls.

At any rate, Valencia clearly stretched the limits of human dehydration well beyond their usual breaking point. And his case offers one additional twist. After a week with no water in furnace-like heat, covering more than a hundred miles on foot, he was very, very thirsty— but he didn't get heatstroke.

No topic of advice in modern sports science has provoked more whiplash than hydration. A century ago, the prevailing advice to endurance athletes was to avoid drinking at all costs. "Don't get in the habit of drinking and eating in a marathon race," warned James E. Sullivan, the author of a 1909 guide to distance running (and the namesake of the award given to the nation's top amateur athlete each year); "some prominent runners do, but it is not beneficial." The logic was that drinking fluids would likely upset your stomach, and wouldn't be absorbed into your system until the race was finished anyway. That advice was still state-of-the-art in 1968, when twenty-one-year-old Amby Burfoot ran the Boston Marathon on a scorching day without drinking anything, losing nearly ten pounds in the process—and won.

But changes were afoot. In 1965, a security guard named Dwayne Douglas at the University of Florida's Health Center was chatting with one of the researchers in the building, who specialized in kidney medicine. Douglas, a former Philadelphia Eagles player and a volunteer assistant with the Gators football team, was puzzled by how much weight his players lost—as much as eighteen pounds, he reported—and the fact that, as he delicately put it, "my football players do not wee wee during the game." The specialist, Robert Cade, was intrigued. He got permission to test players during practices, and eventually came up with a drink containing water, sugar, and salts to replace what the players were losing in sweat (then, when the concoction proved to be undrinkable, added some lemon juice at his wife's suggestion). The head coach allowed Cade to try the drink on his freshman team during an intrasquad scrimmage with the B team—and after being pushed around for two quarters, the well-hydrated freshmen surged to a lead in the second half as the B team wilted. The varsity team used the drink the next day to come back from a 13–0 halftime deficit and eke out a narrow win over heavily favored Louisiana State in 102-degree heat, and the drink that became known as Gatorade never looked back.

It's worth noting that Gatorade isn't just a rehydrator; its sugar also restocks the fuel stores that your muscles are burning through (a topic we'll explore in the next chapter). But the rise of Gatorade kicked off a new era of interest in hydration for athletes, with generously funded research seemingly confirming its importance. A few months before his Boston Marathon win, Burfoot had completed a series of twenty-mile treadmill runs at 6:00-mile pace while drinking water, Gatorade, or nothing—part of the very first external scientific study funded by Gatorade. Many other studies followed, and in 1988 the company established its own Gatorade Sports Science Institute to help spread the message. By 1996, the Gatorade-sponsored American College of Sports Medicine's official position was that athletes should drink early and often in an attempt to "replace all the water lost through sweating . . . or consume the maximal amount that can be tolerated." And it wasn't just athletes: pervasive dehydration was increasingly cast as the hidden scourge of a generation, insidiously robbing children of their vitality and office workers of their cognitive edge.

Then came hyponatremia. The death of twenty-eight-year-old Cynthia Lucero, who collapsed four miles from the finish line of the 2002 Boston Marathon, focused worldwide attention on a problem that had first been identified more than two decades earlier. Though Lucero complained of feeling "dehydrated and rubber-legged" before she collapsed, hospital tests revealed the opposite problem: following the prevailing advice to athletes, she had drunk as much as she could stomach during her run, causing the levels of sodium in her blood to become diluted (that's what "hyponatremia," sometimes referred to as "water intoxication," means). Her lungs filled with fluid, and her brain began to swell, which after a few hours led to her death. Subsequent studies revealed that the condition, though not usually fatal, was showing up in a handful of runners at nearly every major marathon. In 2003, U.S.A. Track and Field rewrote their guidelines to suggest that runners should drink when they're thirsty rather than striving to replace all sweat losses or consuming "the maximal amount that can be tolerated." Other organizations followed, and researchers began to look more closely at the deeply entrenched tenets of conventional wisdom about hydration—with surprising and still-controversial results.

You've heard the warnings. Drink now, because losing just 2 percent of your weight will hurt your performance—and by the time you feel thirsty, it's already too late. This concept of "voluntary dehydration," in which thirst is an inadequate barometer of your fluid needs, dates back to a series of wartime studies led by University of Rochester researcher Edward F. Adolph, which he summarized in a classic 1948 book called *Physiology of Man in the Desert*. With the outbreak of desert warfare in North Africa in 1941, Adolph and his colleagues were dispatched to the Sonoran Desert in California to investigate soldiers' water needs. At the time, there was a widespread belief that you could train yourself to drink less water, which in turn would minimize "wasteful" sweat losses. Adolph and his colleagues debunked this notion and demonstrated that staying hydrated was important even for well-acclimatized desert veterans. But they also made a curious observation: in long desert marches of up to eight hours, even when the men were allowed to drink as much as they pleased, they finished the marches in a state of dehydration, having lost 2 or 3 or sometimes even 4 percent of their starting weight. Tank crews lost an average of 3 percent of their body weight after a few hours of simulated battle; the eight crewmen of a B-17 Flying Fortress returned from a two-hour low-altitude mission having lost 1.6 percent. The logical conclusion, then, was that you need to drink more than you really want to in order to avoid getting dehydrated.

Why should you go to the trouble of drinking more than you want? Adolph's studies suggested that the consequences of dehydration included "generalized discomfort, fatigue, apathy, low morale, and unwillingness and inability to undertake strenuous activity." Then, beginning in the late 1960s, studies (including the one that Amby Burfoot participated in) began to link dehydration more specifically with overheating. It made sense, since dehydration reduces the volume of blood available to shunt heat to your skin, and in extreme cases might even compromise your ability to sweat. The differences in core temperature observed in these studies were subtle, measured in fractions of a degree. Still, hydration—drink as much as you can tolerate—became the go-to advice for preventing heatstroke.

It wasn't just a question of avoiding catastrophes, though. Researchers began to publish findings suggesting that even relatively mild dehydration would hinder both physical and mental performance. A U.S. Army study in 1966 had soldiers walk to exhaustion on an uphill treadmill in a hot room while normally hydrated, dehydrated by 2 percent, or dehydrated by 4 percent. Sure enough, their walking time dropped by an average of 22 percent and 48 percent, respectively, in the two dehydrated trials. Subsequent studies produced similar results, entrenching the familiar "2 percent rule." Put all these findings together—voluntary dehydration, overheating, declining physical performance—and you have a compelling case that even mild dehydration can be debilitating if not dangerous. But that's not the only explanation that fits the observed facts.

Some of the most vivid cautionary tales about dehydration focus on Alberto Salazar, the irascible 1980s marathon star who now coaches an exclusive (and, due to recent accusations of unethical supplement and prescription-medicine use, controversial) squad of some of the world's best runners at Nike headquarters in Oregon. Salazar was famous for his unyielding racing style and his appetite for suffering. As a nineteen-year-old in 1978, he returned home to the Boston suburb of Wayland, Massachusetts, for the summer after a disappointing sixth-place finish at the NCAA championships ended his sophomore track season at the University of Oregon. He made a sign to post on his bedroom wall, scrawled in felt-tip pen on a giant piece of poster board, that he stared at daily: "You will never be broken again."

At the end of that summer, Salazar put this credo into practice at the seven-mile Falmouth Road Race, on Cape Cod, where he lined up against some of the best runners in the world: Bill Rodgers, Craig Virgin, Rudy Chapa. At the four-mile mark, he tried to take the lead. "That's the last thing I remember about the race," Salazar later recalled in his memoir, *14 Minutes*. Witnesses said he stopped, turned around in a circle, then kept running to the finish, where he finished tenth. His next memory is of hearing a series of numbers: "104 . . . 106 . . . 107 . . . it's not going down! I think we're going to lose him!" It was his body temperature: he was submerged in a tub of ice water in the medical tent, suffering from heatstroke, and his life hung in the balance. He was soon rushed to the hospital, where a priest read him his last rites. After an hour, his temperature dropped and he made a full recovery—and if anything, he gained confidence from this seeming confirmation of his toughness.

Four years later, Salazar was the world's preeminent distance runner. He had won the New York Marathon in 1980, while still a student at Oregon, and returned the following year to set a world record of 2:08:13 (though the record was subsequently disallowed due to a course measurement issue). His most famous race, though, remains the 1982 Boston Marathon, a head-to-head battle with upstart rival Dick Beardsley remembered by running fans as the "Duel in the Sun." Boston's noon start meant that the runners faced temperatures in the mid-60s under a cloudless sky, and Salazar drank nearly nothing: perhaps two cups of water in total, just as he had done in his New York triumphs. The two men raced stride for stride for nearly the entire distance, with Salazar edging ahead in the final mile (and Beardsley's late comeback attempt reportedly foiled by the motorcycles and media bus clogging up the finishing straight). Salazar, once again, had to be carted to the medical tent immediately after the finish, where six liters of fluid were pumped intravenously into his twitching body.

Salazar's famous collapses and abstemious hydration habits are still widely cited as evidence of the link between dehydration and heatstroke. But the picture isn't as simple as it seems. In Falmouth, where he undoubtedly ran himself into heatstroke, the race was only 7 miles long—barely more than half an hour—and he was already in trouble shortly after the halfway mark. Salazar was a prodigious sweater (later lab tests showed he could squeeze out an unusually high three liters of sweat per hour), but it's still impossible to get dangerously dehydrated in twenty minutes. Even if he'd been careless about drinking and started the race mildly dehydrated, the math of how much fluid he would have to lose in such a short time simply doesn't add up.

In contrast, he was clearly dehydrated after the Duel in the Sun, and for good reason: he had been pushing himself for more than two hours. The six liters of IV fluid he received suggests he might have lost more than thirteen pounds of sweat during the race. And yet, despite the sun and the excessive dehydration, he didn't suffer from heatstroke. Quite the opposite, in fact: in the medical tent immediately after the race, his body temperature was measured as 88 degrees, 10 degrees *below* normal. This measurement, which was recorded with an oral thermometer, stirred up a tempest among sports medicine doctors after the race. Since it wasn't a core temperature measured in the rectum or ear, skeptics maintained that Salazar wasn't really hypothermic. Instead, they argued, severe dehydration and the associated reduction in blood volume had compromised his body's ability to regulate temperature. William Castelli, the marathon's finish-line medical director (moonlighting from his day job as director of the famously long-running Framingham Heart Study), stuck to his guns: "His arms, hands, and head were cold," he said. "His core may have been warm, but he was shivering and had goose bumps. As far as I'm concerned he was freezing to death." Without a time machine (and a rectal probe), it's impossible to settle the debate one way or the other—but we can rule out heatstroke.

This seemingly contradictory pattern—heatstroke without dehydration, dehydration without heatstroke—is no fluke, it turns out. Dehydration is a greater concern in longer races, because you have more time to sweat; heatstroke, in contrast, is most common in shorter races. That's because your body temperature is primarily determined by your "metabolic rate"—that is, how hot your engine is running. In a thirty-minute race, you can sustain a fast enough pace to drive your core temperature way up, even though you don't have time to get seriously dehydrated. In a three-hour race, in most circumstances, you simply can't sustain a hard enough effort to push your temperature into heatstroke territory, even though you might get seriously dehydrated. It's true that, as early studies like the one Amby Burfoot participated in showed, dehydration can push your temperature up a little bit. But the biggest factor dictating core temperature (aside from the weather conditions) is metabolic rate.

That's why dehydration turned out to be a nonfactor in Jason Stinson's trial. Max Gilpin wasn't dehydrated—but even if he was, it's highly unlikely that drinking more would have made a difference. Unfortunately for Salazar, this turned out to be true for him, too. While preparing for the 1984 Los Angeles Olympics, where conditions for the marathon were expected to be hot and muggy, Salazar worked with a team of scientists at the U.S. Army Research Institute of Environmental Medicine, in Natick, Massachusetts. They put him through heat tolerance tests in a climate chamber, ran blood tests, sent him to Florida with a do-it-yourself rectal thermometer for heat training, and had him drink a liter of water five minutes before the start of the Olympic marathon plus almost two liters during the race itself— a stark contrast to the minimalist approach to hydration he had taken in his record-setting runs in New York and Boston. The result: America's greatest marathon hope struggled to a fifteenth-place finish, almost five minutes behind the winner and six minutes behind his own best time.

More than thirty years after that race, in 2016, I appeared as a guest on an NPR affiliate to talk about the science of hydration. One of the other guests was Lawrence Armstrong, the director of the University of Connecticut's Human Performance Lab, a former president of the American College of Sports Medicine—and the man who had led the U.S. Army team devising Salazar's hydration plan in 1984. It soon became clear that he and I had very different perspectives on the lessons to take from Salazar's experiences. Armstrong still maintained that inadequate hydration is a key risk factor for heatstroke. And he was adamant that losing 2 percent of your body weight inevitably compromises your performance.

But this claim, too, runs into problems when you venture outside the laboratory. On a damp September day in 2007, Ethiopian superstar Haile Gebrselassie surged to a new world record of 2:04:26 at the Berlin Marathon. Like Salazar, Gebrselassie sweats at a prodigious rate: in one lab test, he hit a rate of 3.6 liters per hour, which is among the highest ever recorded. By the end of his world-record run, he had lost nearly 10 percent of his body weight, dropping from 128 to 115.5 pounds. Further in-race measurements of Gebrselassie and other champion marathoners have produced similar results. There are two ways to interpret these data points. Either elite runners like Gebrselassie—whose world record made him the fastest human ever at the marathon distance—run slower than they should because they fail to adhere to the basic hydration advice doled out at every elementary school and fitness club in the world. Or else that familiar advice is wrong.

To my surprise, Armstrong took the former position on the radio show when I brought up the heavy sweat losses of top marathoners: "And I ask, if they did not lose ten pounds, how fast would they run?" When I phoned him later to press him on this point, he offered a more nuanced take. During their pre-Olympic testing in 1984, he and his colleagues had estimated that Salazar's "gastric emptying rate," which determines how much fluid can pass through the stomach for absorption from the small intestine, was about one liter per hour while running. Given that his sweat rate was three times higher than that, there was never any chance he would be able to limit his fluid loss to 2 percent: drinking more would simply leave fluid sloshing around in his stomach without increasing hydration. And since gastric emptying rarely exceeds 1.3 liters per hour, the same is true for many people, meaning that in prolonged exercise in the heat the 2 percent rule is more a theoretical ideal than a realistic plan. Still, Armstrong was adamant that marathoners like Gebrselassie pay a price for the high levels of dehydration they incur. "There is no doubt in my mind that he would run better and faster—no doubt—if he were down around 2 percent instead of 10 percent," he told me.

It's tempting to dismiss Gebrselassie and Salazar as physiological anomalies, which they undoubtedly are. But similar patterns show up in much less rarefied samples. At marathons, triathlons, and cycling races around the world, researchers have tried a simple test: weigh athletes before and after the race, and look for a relationship between race finish and degree of dehydration. The results are consistently the opposite of what you would expect: the fastest finishers tend to be the most dehydrated. For example, among 643 finishers in the 2009 Mont Saint-Michel Marathon in France, sub-three-hour finishers averaged a loss of 3.1 percent of their starting weight; finishers between three and four hours averaged 2.5 percent; and those clocking more than four hours were the only ones to obey the 2 percent rule, losing on average 1.8 percent. The results don't prove that drinking makes you slower, but they certainly raise further questions about the claim that any loss greater than 2 percent slows you down.

As for the relatively common sight of athletes needing assistance or even collapsing after the finish of a long race, there are several reasons to be suspicious of the idea that these athletes are paying the price for insufficient hydration. One is that studies have found no difference between the typical dehydration levels of collapsed athletes and those who walk away from the finish line untroubled. Another is that an estimated 85 percent of collapses take place shortly after crossing the finish line. This suggests that there is something about the act of *stopping* after prolonged exertion that triggers problems; if the cause was dehydration, you would expect to see more athletes crumpling to the pavement in the closing miles of the race rather than a few steps beyond the finish line.

The problem, many researchers now believe, is a loss of blood pressure caused by blood pooling in the legs after you stop running or cycling. During exercise, your heart directs vast quantities of blood to the oxygen-starved muscles in the legs. With each step or pedal stroke, your calf muscles contract and squeeze the blood vessels in the lower leg, helping to mechanically pump this blood back toward the heart. After you cross the finish line, this muscle pump abruptly stops, and in some people circulation doesn't readjust quickly enough to maintain their blood pressure, causing them to feel dizzy or collapse. The solution? At a series of Ironman Triathlons and ultramarathons in South Africa in 2006 and 2007, medical staff randomized collapsed athletes to two possible treatments: those with even-numbered race bibs were given intravenous fluids, which would be the ideal treatment if the underlying problem was dehydration; those with odd-numbered bibs were simply told to lie down and elevate their legs, and allowed to drink as desired. The average time to discharge from the medical tent for both groups was just under an hour, with no statistically significant difference between the two.

How do we reconcile the chasm between the laboratory and real-world effects of dehydration? The first step is to make a distinction between thirst, which is the feeling that you would like to take a drink, and dehydration, which is the state of having lost fluids relative to your normal levels. The World War II–era desert studies make this distinction clear: while being thirsty virtually always indicates that you're dehydrated, the concept of "voluntary dehydration" illustrates that, conversely, being dehydrated won't always make you thirsty. But as Tim Noakes points out, nearly all dehydration studies since then have lumped the two together. Mountains of data now demonstrate that being dehydrated *and* thirsty, even at a relatively mild level, will slow you down. But what if you're in the state of voluntary dehydration, which by definition involves free access to fluids so that you're dehydrated but not thirsty?

To answer that question, it's worth considering what thirst is for. The simplest explanation is that it's the body's way of ensuring that you keep your fluid levels topped up. In this picture, voluntary dehydration is a failure of the system: it indicates that your thirst sensation isn't very good at its job, because it fails to notice that you're losing fluids. But physiologists have shown that this isn't how thirst works. Instead of monitoring fluid levels, your body monitors "plasma osmolality," which is the concentration of small particles like sodium and other electrolytes in your blood. As you get dehydrated, your blood gets more concentrated, and your body responds by secreting an antidiuretic hormone that causes your kidneys to start reabsorbing water, and by making you thirsty. Unlike your body's fluid levels, plasma osmolality is very tightly regulated: when you're looking at the right variable, your thirst sensation (along with other homeostatic mechanisms like antidiuretic hormone) doesn't make mistakes.

This means that what looks like a potential problem—voluntary dehydration—may actually be completely normal from the body's perspective. In a 2011 study, eighteen South African Special Forces soldiers undertook a sixteen-mile march carrying 57-pound packs, including rifles and water supplies, in temperatures that peaked at 112 degrees Fahrenheit. The soldiers were permitted to drink as much water as they wanted, but—as expected—they nonetheless lost an average of six pounds, corresponding to 3.8 percent of their starting weight. Their plasma osmolality, in contrast, was essentially unchanged. From the perspective of the body's primary hydration sensor, they were just fine.

This disconnect between thirst and water loss may actually be an evolutionary advantage rather than a bug. The "born to run" theory of human origins, advanced by evolutionary biologists Dennis Bramble and Daniel Lieberman in 2004, posits that our ability to run long distances over the hot savanna gave us a crucial advantage over other species. To do that, we needed to be able to tolerate temporary periods of dehydration without negative effects, much as the !Xo San Bushman hunter Karoha Langwane did during a 2000 documentary when he hunted a kudu to exhaustion during a twenty-mile chase through the Kalahari Desert. During four to six hours of hunting in temperatures well above 100 degrees, he drank only a liter of water. By adjusting the amount of salt in our sweat, we're able to keep plasma osmolality stable even as we lose water—for a while, at least. Back at the campfire after the hunt is over, we bring our water levels back to normal over the course of several hours.

There's another twist that helps explain how we're able to tolerate seemingly extreme losses of water. In this discussion, we've been assuming that if you lose a pound of weight during exercise, that means you've lost a pound of water. But that's not necessarily the case. In the study of South African soldiers, the volunteers drank a dose of specially prepared "tracer" water before and after the march, in which some of the hydrogen atoms were replaced with deuterium atoms (hydrogen atoms with an extra neutron). This allowed the researchers to accurately measure how much the total amount of water in the body changed during the hike. The results showed that for every pound of weight lost, the amount of water circulating in the body dropped by only 0.2 pounds—a dramatic difference that helps explain why the soldiers didn't feel the need to drink more.

Part of the explanation, according to University of Cape Town researcher Nicholas Tam, is that not all the weight you lose is water. During prolonged exercise, "you will use fat, and you will use carbohydrate," he explains, "and once you've burned it up, it's not there anymore." The chemical reactions involved in burning fat and carbohydrate produce two key by-products: carbon dioxide, which you breathe out, and water—which actually adds to the amount of fluid available in your body. Even more significant, your body stores carbohydrate in your muscles in a form that locks away about three grams of water for every gram of carbohydrate. This water isn't available to contribute to essential cellular processes until you start unlocking the carbohydrate stores, so your body sees it as "new" water when it's released during exercise. For decades, these factors were assumed to be insignificantly small. But in 2007, British scientists at the University of Loughborough estimated that a marathoner could conceivably lose 1 to 3 percent of his or her body mass without any net loss of water. The study with South African soldiers seemed to confirm these estimates, as did a 2011 study by Tam that found no change in total body water content in runners at a half-marathon despite an average weight loss of more than three pounds. The effect is even more pronounced at longer distances: data from the Western States 100-mile race suggests that typical finishers should expect to lose between 4.5 and 6.4 percent of their starting weight just to keep their internal hydration levels steady.

The result is that you can be "dehydrated," at least in the sense that you've lost weight, without hurting your performance. What matters, instead, is how thirsty you are. Unfortunately, virtually all hydration studies since World War II have been designed in a way that makes it impossible to distinguish between dehydration and thirst. Consider, for example, the 1966 U.S. Army study described on page 163, which found that being dehydrated by 2 percent caused a 22 percent decrease in time to exhaustion. To achieve this level of dehydration, the subjects had first walked to exhaustion on a treadmill, then spent six hours confined to a room at 115 degrees to promote sweating—all before even *beginning* their exercise test. Other studies have used diuretics to promote dehydration, and most forbid the subjects from drinking during the bout of exercise. It's not remotely surprising that endurance is reduced under these conditions: in addition to being dehydrated, the subjects are tired, thirsty, and probably pretty annoyed by the whole process.

The more interesting comparison isn't between full hydration and no hydration. It's between drinking as much as you want—enough to abolish thirst, even though you'll still get "voluntarily dehydrated"— and drinking either more or less. That was the goal of a 2009 study at Noakes's lab in Cape Town, in which cyclists completed a series of six fifty-mile time trials. In the first trial, they drank as much as they wanted; in the other five, they were assigned varying levels of hydration ranging from nothing to enough to fully replace all their sweat losses. Sure enough, being hydrated improved performance: in the three trials where the cyclists were forced to drink less than they'd chosen to in the first trial, they were slower than the three higher-hydration trials. But there was no further improvement when they drank *more* than they had chosen to in the first trial. Avoiding thirst, rather than avoiding dehydration, seems to be the most important key to performance.

This controversial claim was mostly dismissed when it was first published, but the debate has gradually shifted in the years since then. A 2013 meta-analysis in the *British Journal of Sports Medicine* concluded than any losses of less than 4 percent are "very unlikely to impair [endurance performance] under real-world exercise conditions," and concluded that athletes should be encouraged to drink according to thirst.

Still, as compelling as these lines of evidence are, focusing on the details of plasma osmolality and total body water misses a larger point that has recurred throughout this book: the importance of any underlying physiological signal depends in part on how your brain receives and interprets it. "When you drink, you're also affecting your thirst, your perception, your psychology, your motivation," says Stephen Cheung, the Brock University cyclist and environmental physiologist we met in the previous chapter. If you're stuck in an uncomfortable heat chamber and told you'll only be allowed to drink a few thimblefuls of water, your performance will likely suffer whether you're dehydrated or not. To get around this problem, Cheung decided to try hydrating a group of cyclists intravenously. The study was double-blinded, meaning that neither the subjects nor the researchers knew how dehydrated a cyclist was allowed to get during each ride; instead, a paramedic hidden behind a curtain controlled how much (if any) saline solution was infused into their arms. The results showed that, in a twenty-kilometer time trial following ninety minutes of steady riding in the heat, even 3 percent dehydration had no effect on performance.

Other studies have shown that the mere act of swallowing fluids— a feeling the cyclists in Cheung's study were denied—effectively fights thirst and improves performance. A famous 1997 study at Yale had subjects exercise for two hours to induce dehydration, then allowed them to drink and monitored the changes in perceived thirst and antidiuretic hormone, the two key regulators of plasma osmolality. Then they repeated the trial, but inserted a tube down through the nose into the stomach to vacuum out the water as soon as it was swallowed. The result: thirst and antidiuretic hormone secretion both decreased anyway, presumably in response to the sensation of water flowing down the throat. And when they reversed the experiment, sending the same amount of water *down* the nasogastric tube instead of letting the subjects swallow it, it was less effective in quenching thirst even though the water was allowed to stay in their stomachs.

This, in turn, helps to explain why a later study found that swallowing small mouthfuls of water—too small to make any difference to overall hydration levels—boosted exercise performance by 17 percent compared to rinsing the same amount of water in the mouth and then spitting it out. When it comes to quenching your thirst, perception— not just in your mouth, but in the cool flow of liquid down a parched throat—is, at least in part, reality.

So is dehydration really a vast corporate conspiracy whose effects are all in your head (or throat)? Not quite. In recent years, the debate about hydration has become increasingly polarized. Gadflies like Tim Noakes have at times seemed to argue that hydration doesn't matter at all: in his 2012 book, *Waterlogged*, he somewhat facetiously suggested that true dehydration in marathon runners should be diagnosed by the signs observed in a company of U.S. cavalrymen who got lost in the Texas desert in 1877: "an uncontrollable desire for water; inability to detect the presence of fluid or food in the mouth; inability to masticate food; uncontrollable desire to ingest any fluid, even blood or urine." That seems a little extreme. Meanwhile, respected establishment voices like Lawrence Armstrong continue to maintain that thirst is a completely inadequate guide to hydration and that even the mildest loss of fluids will cause trouble.

For a middle ground between these two perspectives, I've found that the physiologists who work with Olympic athletes are often best at reconciling abstract theory with the cold, hard practice of elite sport. "Anyone who has worked in the field with athletes has probably realized years ago that a strict two-percent dehydration cut-off just doesn't work," says Trent Stellingwerff, a physiologist at the Canadian Sport Institute Pacific, in Victoria, British Columbia. In his work with elite marathoners, Stellingwerff aims for 3 to 6 percent dehydration, depending on weather and individual tolerance. Simply drinking to thirst doesn't cut it for elite marathoners, because drinks are only available every 5K or so, and the jostling motion of fast running makes it difficult to drink as much as they would otherwise choose.

Even Haile Gebrselassie, who set world records while losing 10 percent of his body weight, didn't rely on a "drink when you feel like it" plan. That's what he tried in his very first marathon, in 2002, when he pressed the pace early on but eventually blew up and was passed by rivals Khalid Khannouchi and Paul Tergat. In later—and more successful—marathons, he followed a carefully planned hydration strategy. During his 2007 world-record race in Berlin, according to Stellingwerff, Gebrselassie's plan involved a bottle of sports drink three hours before the race, another one an hour before the race, and then a total of two liters of water and sports drink during the race, consumed at 5K intervals. He wasn't following the 2 percent rule, but he was certainly following a premeditated drinking plan.

One final caveat is that our ability to tolerate temporary bouts of dehydration is, well, temporary. Marathoners can handle 10 percent dehydration for a few hours. But that assumes you're properly hydrated when you arrive at the start line—a factor that is, if anything, even more important than what you drink during exercise, according to Stephen Cheung's research. And what if you're doing an Ironman triathlon, or grueling multi-day ultra like the sixty-hour Barkley Marathons, far beyond the evolutionary template that presumably shaped our sense of thirst? The short answer is: we don't know. And in the absence of evidence, it makes sense to err on the side of caution and minimize dehydration (not just thirst) during extremely prolonged bouts of exercise. When I go for week-long backcountry hikes in the mountains (or, for that matter, one-hour trail runs in the unpopulated desert parkland near my in-laws' place in Tucson), I know that the consequences of any errors are so severe that it's better to "stay ahead of thirst."

The overturning of conventional wisdom on hydration has been so rapid and confusing that you now hear people arguing that staying hydrated is actually *bad*. After all, the thinking goes, if Haile Gebrselassie loses twelve pounds during a marathon, it makes him that much lighter and faster. Some scientists have made similar arguments about cycling in the mountains, where the benefits of staying light might exceed the benefits of staying hydrated.

I'm not convinced by these arguments. To me, the primary message is that, like oxygen and heat and (as we'll discover) fuel, the loss of fluids first makes itself felt via the brain. Thirst, not dehydration, increases your sense of perceived effort and in turn causes you to slow down. Eventually, the physiological consequences of dehydration assert themselves, increasing the strain on your cardiovascular system and pushing your core temperature up as the volume of blood in your arteries decreases. But that only happens if you've already ignored the signs of thirst.

That means that hydration still matters. Stephen Cheung, for example, still takes two full water bottles along on long bike rides, despite the results of his IV study. It's just not as imminent a crisis as we've been led to believe—and this finding has implications. Cheung points to the disappointing performance of American cyclist Taylor Phinney after he dropped a water bottle at the world championships in 2013. The race was only an hour long, so it shouldn't have mattered—but since Phinney believed it was a problem, it hurt his ride. That's the message Cheung hopes people will take from his study, and from the spate of recent research challenging hydration orthodoxy: not that you shouldn't drink when you have the chance, but that you shouldn't obsess about it when you don't. "It's one less psychological crutch," he says, "to hold you back from a top performance."

CHAPTER 10

Fuel

The meals themselves didn't seem that unusual. For breakfasts, Olympic racewalker Evan Dunfee and his training partners would fill up on muesli with cream or bacon and eggs; lunches featured sandwiches with low-carb bread and lots of avocado; and dinners, specially prepared by the chefs at the Australian Institute of Sport and measured to the ounce for each athlete, ranged from almond satay or zucchini pasta to plain old pizza and burgers. This was the easy part of the diet. "Before and during training was where things got weird," says Dunfee. Before a grueling twenty-five-mile workout, he would fuel up with two boiled eggs and some nutballs: "nuts, cocoa, and I'm not sure what else to hold them together," he recalls, "but they were alright." For mid-workout fueling, instead of gels and sports drink, it was peanut butter cookies and cheese.

The diet was a radical departure for Dunfee, a twenty-five-year-old Canadian from Vancouver, and a risk—it was less than nine months before the 2016 Olympics in Rio, where he hoped to contend for a medal. But elite racewalkers are . . . different. The event, which requires walking as quickly as possible while straightening your leg with each stride and keeping one foot on the ground at all times, is often the butt of jokes, both for its distinctive swivel-hipped stride and for its fundamental premise: NBC sports commentator Bob Costas famously compared it to a contest to see who can whisper the loudest. As a result, top racewalkers from around the world form a notably cohesive clique, even though they're fierce rivals on the tarmac. "This is largely forced upon us," Dunfee says, "as we're usually the most marginalized of all event groups." Still, it meant that Dunfee was receptive when Australian walker Jared Tallent, the defending Olympic champion in the 50-kilometer event, approached him about the possibility of skipping the boreal winter and instead flying south to train in Australia, where he would take part in an unprecedented study of a radical sports nutrition scheme that was generating buzz and controversy in equal measures: low-carbohydrate, high-fat, or "LCHF" diets.

The LCHF debate, which has been roiling the weight-loss world since the early 2000s, had recently made the leap to endurance sport. At first it was a few maverick scientists and would-be gurus; then some long-haired, dogma-defying ultra-runners; then, suddenly, Tim Noakes himself, author of the most influential running book of all time, embraced the cause with his customary fervor. "For 33 years I followed and advocated through my book, *Lore of Running*, the current dogma that to be active and healthy, one must eat a diet low in fat and high in carbohydrate," he wrote in 2015. "I now believe that this advice was quite wrong. I apologize. It was an honest error."

In Canberra, the staid government town where the Australian Institute of Sport's manicured playing fields and high-tech labs are located, Dunfee and Tallent were joined by nineteen other world-class racewalkers from five different continents for the LCHF study, code-named "Supernova." While in residence at the AIS, the walkers followed a standardized training plan, and for periods of three weeks at a time, they adhered to strictly controlled diets that either followed conventional sports nutrition advice for endurance athletes (60 to 65 percent of calories from carbohydrate, 15 to 20 percent from protein, and 20 percent from fat) or an extreme LCHF diet (75 to 80 percent fat, 15 to 20 percent protein, and less than 50 grams per day of carbohydrate—the equivalent of two small bananas). Before and after the three-week diets, the athletes gave samples of blood and poop, completed a series of treadmill tests in the lab, and put their hard-earned fitness to the only test that really matters: a race.

For Dunfee, the transition to LCHF was rocky. In his first fully carb-free workout, what should have been an easy 30-kilometer walk in two and a half hours turned into a "death march," and he actually collapsed at the finish. Later that week, he set an all-time personal worst with his slowest 10-kilometer walk ever. Subsequent weeks went a little better, but his heart rate was consistently higher than usual during training, and so was his sense of effort. At the end of three weeks, lab testing showed that he was measurably less efficient, and he was slower in his 10-kilometer race. Overall, the results seemed disappointing. So it was with a palpable sense of relief that he resumed his standard high-carbohydrate diet. Almost immediately, he felt better and began crushing his workouts. Just ten days later, he headed to Melbourne for a race—where, to everyone's surprise, he shattered the Canadian 50-kilometer walk record with a time of 3:43:45, establishing himself as a podium contender for Rio.

When your car runs out of gas, it stops. In a very simplified sense, your body behaves in the same way. The fuel you use is supplied by food, which contains energy stored in the form of chemical bonds between atoms; those bonds are broken as the food is metabolized, releasing energy that powers your muscles and other organs. If you completely run out of food energy, of course, a bad race is the least of your worries. The records for longest survival without food are both grim and confusing, depending on the precise circumstances and the trustworthiness of the witnesses. A frequently cited benchmark is Kieran Doherty, an Irish Republican Army prisoner at the infamous Maze Prison near Belfast, who refused food for 73 days in 1981 before dying. If you bend the rules a bit to allow vitamins in addition to water, then you'll be able to continue accessing your body's fat stores for much longer. A 1973 journal article by a Scottish doctor reports the case of A.B., a twenty-seven-year-old man who weighed 456 pounds before undertaking a medically supervised fast lasting 382 days, during which he lost a remarkable 276 pounds.

Such feats show that, no matter how badly you bonk during your Ironman, your gas tank isn't truly empty. In fact, performance starts declining long before the needle hits E, for reasons that aren't always obvious. In one study that launched a thousand maternal I-told-you-sos, British researchers found that skipping breakfast resulted in a 4.5 percent drop in 30-minute cycling time trial performance at 5 P.M. that afternoon, even though the subjects had been allowed to eat as much as they wanted at lunch. On a longer time scale, researchers at the University of Minnesota put thirty-six men—all conscientious objectors who had chosen alternative forms of service during World War II—through a twelve-week period of semi-starvation during which their daily calorie intake was cut in half and they lost roughly a quarter of their body weight. Their endurance, measured by an uphill treadmill test to exhaustion with two technicians positioned behind the machine to catch their crumpled bodies, dropped by 72 percent by the end of the experiment. One man lasted just nineteen seconds in the final treadmill test.

It's not just how much fuel is in the tank, in other words. Endurance performance also depends on what types of fuel you have available, where it's stored, and how quickly you can access it. The three basic fuel options are protein, carbohydrate, and fat. While protein is important for building and repairing muscles after resistance exercise, it plays a negligible role in directly fueling muscle contractions. (That said, when you're running low on other sources of fuel during an extended effort, protein can contribute up to 10 percent of your fuel needs—which means that, contrary to popular dogma, even skinny endurance athletes do need more protein than the average nonathlete.) For the most part, though, carbohydrate and fat stoke the furnace during prolonged exercise—and their relative importance has been debated for more than a century.

Early experiments in the first half of the twentieth century showed that the balance between fat and carbohydrate use depends on how hard you're working. During easy exercise, like a gentle walk, you burn mostly fat from the supplies circulating in your bloodstream. As you speed up, you begin to add more carbohydrate to the mix, and by the time you're panting heavily, the proportions have flipped and you're burning mostly carbohydrate. The precise blend depends on a variety of factors: the fitter you are, for example, the greater the proportion of fat you burn at any given speed. (That's simply because maintaining a given speed gets easier as you get fitter. As John Hawley, an exercise metabolism researcher at Australian Catholic University, points out, no matter how fit you are you'll burn the same fat-carb mix at any given *relative* intensity.) Eating a diet high in either fat or carbohydrate also tilts your preferred fuel mix in that direction. But even taking these factors into account, carbohydrates dominate for any intense exercise: one study found that over the marathon distance, running at 2:45 pace relied on 97 percent carbohydrate fuel, while slowing down to 3:45 pace reduced the carbohydrate mix to 68 percent.

The cliché of the pasta-fueled marathoner can be traced back to the work of Swedish scientists Jonas Bergström and Eric Hultman in 1960s. Bergström pioneered the use of needle biopsies, a technique that allowed researchers to slice out small pieces of muscle from their long-suffering research volunteers—or, as was the habit in Scandinavian labs at the time, from their own muscles. In one notable study, Bergström and Hultman sat on opposite sides of a stationary bike, each pedaling with one leg while the other leg rested, until they were both too exhausted to continue. Self-inflicted muscle biopsies before and after cycling showed that levels of glycogen, the form in which carbohydrate is stored in muscles, had dropped to zero in the exercised leg. Running out of this specific muscle fuel, in other words, seemed to coincide with exhaustion. Over the next three days, the two men ate a high-carbohydrate diet and performed regular biopsies. Glycogen levels stayed roughly constant in their rested legs, but in the exercised legs, levels shot up to twice their initial value—a supercompensation effect that launched the idea of "carbohydrate loading" before long-distance races.

Subsequent biopsy studies confirmed that the amount of glycogen you can stuff into your muscles is a pretty good predictor of how long you'll last on a treadmill or stationary bike test to exhaustion. There are other sources of carbohydrate in the body; your liver, for example, can store 400 or 500 calories of glycogen for use throughout the body, compared to about 2,000 for fully loaded leg muscles. (That's why it's useful to eat a small breakfast a few hours before a morning marathon: while your muscles remain fully stocked, your liver glycogen gets depleted because it fuels your energy-hungry brain while you sleep.) Your muscles can also dip into the glucose circulating in your blood, though the total amount of glucose in circulation at any given moment is very small. Overall, the picture that emerged from these studies is relatively simple, harking back to A. V. Hill's "human body as a machine" view: you can store a finite amount of carbohydrate fuel in your body, and when you use it up, you bonk.

If that's the case, then it makes sense for endurance athletes to stock up on carbohydrates as much as possible. And that, more or less, is what sports nutritionists have been advocating since the 1970s. Keep your glycogen levels high by consuming a diet that gets 60 to 65 percent of its calories from carbohydrate; top up your stores by carbo-loading in the final few days before a competition; and in events lasting longer than about ninety minutes, eat or drink some easily digested carbohydrates to supplement your stored glycogen, which will otherwise run out. (Modern sports nutrition guidelines, Hawley points out, actually recommend a daily target amount of carbohydrate per pound of total body weight based on the type of training you've done that day, rather than overall percentage targets. This helps account for the considerable differences between the needs of, say, an elfin distance runner and a heavyweight rower.) Empirically speaking, this advice seems to work pretty well. One study found that Kenyan runners, who currently hold 60 of the top 100 men's marathon times in history, typically get 76.5 percent of their calories from carbohydrate, including 23 percent from ugali, a sticky and stomach-filling cornmeal mash, and 20 percent from the copious spoonfuls of sugar they heap into their tea and porridge. Another 35 times on the top-100 list are held by Ethiopians; a similar study found that they get 64.3 percent of their calories from carbohydrate, with the biggest contribution from injera, a sourdough flatbread made from a local grain called teff. If there's an alternative diet plan that's better for endurance performance, no one has told the best endurance athletes in the world.

On April 1, 1879, Frederick Schwatka and his companions set out across the Arctic tundra from their camp on the northwestern shores of Hudson Bay. Schwatka had been sent north by the American Geographical Society to search for traces of the lost Franklin expedition, which had disappeared three decades earlier while searching for the Northwest Passage, with the presumed loss of 129 men. Schwatka's team, in contrast, was tiny: he had just three companions, and they hired an Inuit guide and three sled drivers, along with their wives and children, to accompany them. The group set off with three sleds pulled by forty-four dogs, weighed down by nearly four thousand pounds of walrus meat for the dogs plus bundles of hard bread, pork, corned beef, and other supplies. In total, the rations were expected to last for about a month. By the time they returned to their base camp, 11 months and 20 days later, they had covered a record-setting 3,251 miles by sled, while enduring temperatures that over one three-month period *averaged* –50 degrees Fahrenheit; located some telling remains of Franklin's expedition (including further evidence that some of the men had resorted to cannibalism); discovered new rivers and other geographical features; and suffered not a single casualty.

Much as, a century later, the nimble alpine-style ascents of Reinhold Messner represented a break from the cumbersome military-style expeditions that were then standard in mountaineering, Schwatka's trip helped to usher in a new style of exploration. Franklin's epic debacle was by no means an isolated incident. Across the globe, European explorers were trying to bulldoze their way into remote and unfamiliar environments with spectacularly inappropriate equipment and ill-considered plans. In Australia, for example, the Burke and Wills expedition of 1860 set off into the country's arid interior at the height of summer, with twenty-three horses and twenty-six camels toting a ridiculous load including "a Chinese gong, a stationary cabinet, [and] a heavy wooden table with matching stools." Like Franklin, Burke and Wills ended up dying of starvation in a region that, to those who lived there, seemed abundantly supplied with food.

Schwatka had no experience in the Arctic, but he was a careful and capable leader who had gained respect for the traditional knowledge of native people during his service as a cavalry officer in the American west. While in the army, he also managed to find time to qualify as both a lawyer and, a year later, a doctor. "And he possesses a very important adjunct, though to the uninitiated it may seem trifling," one of his trip-mates reported: "a stomach that can relish and digest fat." Schwatka's decision to carry only a month of food meant that he and his companions would have to live off the land, as the Inuit in the region did. That meant a diet that, for much of the year, consisted of nothing but fish and meat—a sure recipe, you would think, for diseases of deficiency like scurvy and for a general lack of carbohydrate-powered energy for physical exertion.

In the end, the men killed and ate a total of 522 reindeer during their trip, plus muskoxen, polar bears, and seals. For one two-week period, they ate nothing but ducks. Adapting to the diet took time: "When first thrown wholly upon the diet of reindeer meat, it seems inadequate to properly nourish the system and there is an apparent weakness and inability to perform severe exertive, fatiguing journeys," Schwatka noted in his diary. "But this soon passes away in the course of 2-3 weeks." After close to a year of rigorous travel on this diet, he was as fit as ever, capable of walking 65 miles in two days to meet the whaling ship that would take him home.

Schwatka's adventure should have debunked once and for all the myth that the Inuit had some unique evolutionary powers that enabled them to survive for much of the year on meat alone. But that aspect of his journey was mostly overlooked until a later explorer and anthropologist, Vilhjalmur Stefansson, reached similar conclusions in the early 1900s. Stefansson left a post at Harvard to join an expedition to the

Arctic, where through a series of mishaps he found himself stranded for the winter alone with a group of Inuit, forced to rely on their hospitality—and on their diet, which consisted of raw, half-frozen fish for breakfast and lunch, and boiled fish for dinner. Stefansson didn't even like fish, but out of necessity he soon adapted. He eventually ventured to try the rotten fish kept from the previous summer, which was considered a special delicacy—and, to his surprise, "liked it better than my first taste of Camembert."

In subsequent expeditions, Stefansson insisted that he and his men eat Inuit-style, and he spent a total of more than five years living on fish, meat, and water. His dietary claims were so controversial that he and a fellow explorer eventually agreed to spend a year living on an all-meat diet in New York under close medical supervision, funded by the Institute of American Meat Packers. The results, which were published in 1930 in the *Journal of Biological Chemistry,* generally supported his claims of good health. Neither man developed scurvy, thanks to the vitamin C contained in animal organs and other cuts. Stefansson's worst moments came at the start of the experiment, when the investigators fed him only lean meat. In the Arctic, he had noted, the Inuit relished the fattiest parts of the animal, giving the leanest meat to the dogs. Once he switched to fattier cuts, so that about three-quarters of his calories came from fat, he was fine. Every few weeks, the two explorers were led on a run around the Central Park reservoir and then subjected to a series of tests to assess their stamina, which appeared to improve as the experiment wore on.

Proving that you can survive on meat alone—as remarkable as that still seems—is different than proving it's a *superior* diet, and in particular that it enhances endurance. Stefansson continued to advocate for the benefits of a high-fat meat diet, including suggesting during World War II that troops should be outfitted with emergency rations of pemmican, a hearty mix of dried meat and rendered fat that native Canadians and northern explorers had relied on for generations. But when the proposal was put to the test by a platoon of seasoned troops during a simulated subarctic combat mission, the results, published in 1945 in the journal *War Medicine,* were disastrous: "Morale fell abruptly on the first day of pemmican diet and by the second day excessive fatigue, weakness, and nausea appeared. On the third day the platoon had deteriorated beyond the point of military usefulness. Vomiting and exhaustion compelled the officers in charge to terminate the test."

This failure, combined with other studies that found superior endurance on high-carbohydrate diets compared to low-carbohydrate diets, helped put LCHF on the back burner for athletes and scientists. There were some caveats, though, as a medical researcher at the Massachusetts Institute of Technology named Stephen Phinney pointed out in 1983. For one thing, as Schwatka had found, it takes several weeks for the body to adjust to a mostly carbohydrate-free diet—longer than any of the failed studies had allowed. The studies also didn't ensure adequate salt intake, which Phinney believed was crucial, and they sometimes conflated "high fat" with "high protein." While most of us intuitively think of an all-meat diet as being high in protein, an ounce of fat contains more than twice as many calories as an ounce of protein. Phinney put five well-trained cyclists on a diet modeled after Stefansson's, with 83 percent of the calories from fat, 15 percent from protein, and just 2 percent from carbohydrate, for four weeks. The results, which have acquired near-scriptural status in the LCHF community, showed that the cyclists' VO_2max and performance in a multi-hour time-to-exhaustion test remained essentially unchanged. In other words, with enough adaptation time, you could apparently run your engine on fat just as well as it runs on carbohydrate.

For sports scientists, this was an enticing prospect. As we've seen, a well-prepared athlete might be able to store 2,500 calories of carbohydrate; running a marathon, for a 150-pound runner, takes around 3,000 calories, most of which will come from carbohydrate if you're racing as fast as you can. That means you either need to refuel along the route, which carries its own set of challenges, or slow down. Meanwhile, whether you like it or not, you're lugging at least 30,000 (and for most of us closer to 100,000) calories of fat with you. If, like Phinney's cyclists, you could access those fat stores while exercising at a moderately high intensity, you could keep going long enough that sleep deprivation would be a bigger problem than bonking.

In practice, though, there were some important caveats. With just five subjects, Phinney's results were highly variable: one subject improved his time to exhaustion from 148 to 232 minutes, while another declined from 140 to 89 minutes. And there was a crucial trade-off, Phinney acknowledged: in exchange for their enhanced ability to burn fat, the cyclists seemed to have lost some of their ability to harness quick-burning carbohydrate for short sprints, resulting in "a severe restriction on the ability of subjects to do anaerobic work."

Over the next few decades, as sports scientists around the world experimented with various fat-adaptation protocols, they ran into this problem over and over. Finally, a definitive 2005 study at the University of Cape Town (coauthored by subsequent LCHF convert Tim Noakes) put cyclists through a 100-kilometer time trial that incorporated five 1-kilometer sprints and four 4-kilometer sprints, in an attempt to simulate the thrust and parry of hill climbs and breakaways during a Tour de France stage. Once again, overall performance in the time trial was unchanged on a high-fat diet, but sprint performance—the moments, in cycling, where races are won and lost—was compromised. In an accompanying commentary, Louise Burke, the head of sports nutrition at the Australian Institute of Sport and one of the leading researchers on fat-adaptation protocols, pronounced the study the "nail in the coffin" for high-fat diets as a performance booster. The following year, Trent Stellingwerff, then a Ph.D. student at the University of Guelph, showed why: high-fat diets don't just ramp up fat burning; they actually throttle carbohydrate usage by decreasing the activity of a key enzyme called pyruvate dehydrogenase.

The role that fuel stores play in the limits of endurance depends, of course, on what we mean by endurance. If you're simply concerned with covering the greatest distance possible, without a particular focus on time or outsprinting rivals, then you might not care about pyruvate dehydrogenase. And in particular, if you're in a situation when your ability to eat is severely constrained—an expedition across the Antarctic, for example, or a multi-day ultra-race where you can eat only what you carry—then the ability to tap into fat stores seems like a considerable advantage. The bigger the gas tank, the farther you can go and the less you need to refuel.

But if your view of endurance involves racing—squeezing as much distance as possible out of the unforgiving minute—then it turns out that your primary fuel-related concern is not how much but rather how fast. How quickly do your muscles burn fuel? How quickly can they access the various sources of fuel scattered throughout your body? And how quickly can you refill those reservoirs as you go?

In the last chapter, I described the hydration plan that Haile Gebrselassie used when he set a world record of 2:04:26 at the Berlin Marathon in 2007, which involved drinking about two liters of fluid during the race. In practice, his plan was as much focused on fueling as on hydration. Of the two liters of fluid he planned to consume during the race, 1.25 L was sports drink (the rest was water), and he also took five sports gels, providing a total of between 60 and 80 grams of carbohydrate per hour. That number is significant, because scientists have traditionally figured that 60 grams an hour (about 250 calories) is pretty much the maximum amount you can absorb during exercise. The rate-limiting step is the absorption of carbohydrate from the intestine into the bloodstream.

But Gebrselassie was taking advantage of newly published (at the time) data showing that if you combine two different types of carbohydrate—glucose and fructose, for example—they pass through the intestinal wall using two different cellular routes that can operate simultaneously, enabling you to absorb as much as 90 grams of carbohydrate per hour. Stomaching that much carbohydrate in the middle of a race is no easy task—that's why Nike's two-hour-marathon scientists spent so much time trying to help their athletes, particularly Zersenay Tadese and Lelisa Desisa, increase the amount they could stomach during training runs. The Nike team also mixed various drinks together to find personalized carbohydrate combinations that would maximize palatability and absorption rate for each runner. For the rest of us, glucose-fructose mixes are now incorporated in standard sports drinks from companies like PowerBar and Gatorade. If you can stomach more than 60 grams per hour, the higher absorption rate should help stave off the depletion of your glycogen stores and allow you to maintain a faster pace for longer without hitting the wall.

In theory, the math behind this sort of fueling plan is simple: the number of calories you need to ingest is the difference between how many you already have stored in your body and how many you want to burn. In practice, though, the body's workings turn out to be considerably more complicated. Researchers in Scandinavia have recently shown that glycogen stores in your muscles don't just act as energy reservoirs; they also help individual muscle fibers contract efficiently. That means your muscles will weaken as you burn through your glycogen stores, sapping your strength long before you're actually out of fuel. In effect, your muscles have a cunning self-defense mechanism that's totally independent of the brain, the equivalent of having your car's maximum speed linked to the level of its fuel gauge. Moreover, they'll preferentially burn some of the glycogen within the muscle before turning to glucose from your bloodstream—which means, in practical terms, that all the Gatorade in the world won't stave off fatigue indefinitely.

In other ways, though, sports drinks are surprisingly—almost inexplicably—effective. If your body can store enough carbohydrate for 90 minutes or more of exercise, why do some studies find subtle performance boosts from sports drinks in exercise bouts lasting as little as half an hour? And moreover, why do those boosts kick in pretty much instantaneously, long before the carbohydrates have even left your stomach? The easy answer is that the benefits are all in your head—that it's a placebo effect. But that's only partially correct.

A series of studies by Asker Jeukendrup, the sports nutrition researcher who led the development of glucose-fructose mixtures, found that glucose-based sports drink boosted performance in a one-hour cycling time trial. But when, instead of drinking a glucose drink, the cyclists had glucose infused directly into their bloodstream—which should have been *more* effective—the benefits disappeared. So, in 2004, Jeukendrup and his colleagues tried a different approach: this time they asked the cyclists to swish the sports drink in their mouths and then spit it out without swallowing. It worked: simply having sports drink in your mouth seemed to be more important than getting it into your bloodstream and to your muscles. It's important to note that these studies were placebo-controlled: the drinks all tasted the same. Still, it's hard to shake the feeling that a placebo effect must have crept in, and many scientists remained skeptical of the findings.

It wasn't until 2009 that researchers at the University of Birmingham settled the debate, with a study that confirmed the performance benefits of swishing and spitting a carbohydrate drink—and used functional magnetic resonance imaging to show that brain areas associated with reward were lighting up as soon as the subjects had carbohydrate in their mouth. Crucially, neither the brain scan nor cycling performance showed any effects when the drink was artificially sweetened, but the benefits returned when maltodextrine, a tasteless and undetectable carbohydrate, was added to the artificially sweetened drink. The sweet taste of sugar, in other words, is not enough to trigger the benefits. Instead, the mouth appears to contain previously unknown (and as yet unidentified) sensors that relay the presence of carbohydrate directly to the brain. In Tim Noakes's central governor framework, it's as if the brain relaxes its safety margin when it knows (or is tricked into believing) that more fuel is on the way.

The results explain why carbohydrate offers a boost more or less instantaneously, and why studies have found improved performance in efforts as short as half an hour. And there's a further wrinkle that shows just how sophisticated the brain's control mechanism is: the effectiveness of carbohydrate drinks depend on how hungry or well fueled you are. In one 2015 study, Brazilian researchers had cyclists complete a series of 20-kilometer time trials under three conditions: fed (6 A.M. breakfast, 8 A.M. time trial); fasted (no breakfast prior to 8 A.M. time trial); or depleted (like fasted, but with a workout the previous evening followed by a low-carbohydrate dinner). Rinsing and spitting sports drink produced the biggest benefit in the depleted condition, a smaller benefit in the fasted condition, and none at all in the fed condition. Other studies have found similar patterns for swallowing sports drinks in events shorter than about 90 minutes: it only helps if your body is low on fuel to start with.

In practice, these findings mean that the benefits of sports drinks and other mid-race carbohydrates for short bouts of exercise are irrelevant as long as you don't start out with an empty stomach and depleted fuel stores. (Pro tip: you shouldn't.) On a more theoretical level, the results are among the strongest evidence we have that your brain is looking out for your well-being in ways that are outside your conscious control and that kick in long before you reach a point of actual physiological crisis.

By 2013, when *Men's Journal* ran a much-circulated article about elite endurance athletes who had "pushed away the time-honored plate of pasta in favor of . . . copious amounts of healthy fat," the LCHF diet had become a full-fledged trend in the ultra-running community despite the continued skepticism of sports nutritionists. It's not hard to see why: the loss of sprint power on LCHF demonstrated by Phinney and explained by Stellingwerff isn't a big deal for most ultra-runners, who are more interested in completing the distance than in hitting a specific time or outsprinting a rival. In races that last 12 or 20 or—like the infamous Barkley Marathons in Tennessee—60 hours, even the fastest competitors can't sustain the kind of high-intensity pace that burns pure carbohydrate anyway, so fat-burning capacity is already an important part of the metabolic equation. Moreover, one of the biggest challenges for ultra-runners is refueling: convincing your recalcitrant stomach to accept yet another sports gel or banana or whatever else you're trying to force down your gullet after twelve hours on the trail, without sending you scurrying to the bushes. Anything that reduces your dependence on external carbohydrates, and allows you to instead rely on the steady flame of your internal fat stores, has the potential to help. Similar arguments won converts in other longer-than-marathon disciplines like Ironman triathlon and endurance cycling.

To see just how much of a difference high-fat diets could make, a team led by Jeff Volek of Ohio State University (and including LCHF pioneer Stephen Phinney) recruited twenty elite ultra-runners and Ironman triathletes, half of whom had voluntarily switched to an LCHF diet months or years earlier, and brought them to the lab for testing. The results, published in the journal *Metabolism* in 2016, showed that the fat-adapted runners were able to burn fat twice as quickly as the non-fat-adapted control group. During a three-hour treadmill run at a moderate pace, they relied on fat for 88 percent of their energy, compared to 56 percent for those following a standard carbohydrate-heavy diet. That last number is worth noting: even on a high-carbohydrate diet, you still have access to your fat stores during exercise. But the LCHF runners were pushing this ability to a new, previously unseen level: "The rates of fat burning are extraordinary based on conventional wisdom," Volek says.

Still, few of the new converts to LCHF were doing the full Schwatka with more than 80 percent fat and virtually no carbohydrate. Zach Bitter, who set a U.S. track 100-mile record in 2015, and Timothy Olson, who set a course record at the Western States 100-miler in 2012 (and was one of the athletes featured in the 2013 *Men's Journal* article), both say they keep overall carbohydrate intake low but ramp it up before and during long training runs and races. Olson, for example, eats sweet potatoes the night before long runs and takes in one or two gels per hour (each with 100 calories of carbohydrate) during races.

The other two athletes cited in the *Men's Journal* article turn out to have similarly moderate dietary habits. The "high-fat" diet followed by two-time Olympic triathlon medalist Simon Whitfield, for example, turns out be about 50 percent carbohydrate, 30 percent protein, and just

20 percent fat—not exactly skim milk and egg whites, but still closer to standard sports nutrition guidelines than to LCHF territory. And Tour de France cyclist Dave Zabriskie, when I contacted him to ask about his LCHF experience, said that the experiment was interesting but hardly performance-enhancing: "For long easy training, it's good. For day-after-day racing like the Tour, you have to eat the carbs."

To judge from the polarized debate on Internet forums and social media networks, you might think you have to pick a side: you either burn fat or carbohydrate, and woe to you if you make the wrong choice. In reality, as Volek's data shows, we all use both. And given the complementary strengths and weaknesses of the two options—carbohydrate as a fast fuel with limited storage capability, fat as an inexhaustible but rate-limited alternative, it makes sense to aim for what Louise Burke, of the Australian Institute of Sport, calls "metabolic flexibility," by maximizing both fuel pathways. That, in effect, is what ultra-runners like Bitter and Olson are aiming for when they add targeted carbohydrate use before and during key workouts and races, while keeping overall fat levels high. And a mirror image of that approach—a standard high-carbohydrate diet while starting a few workouts each week with deliberately depleted carbohydrate stores—is what Burke and many other researchers around the world pursued in the years after she pronounced the "nail in the coffin" for high-fat diets in 2006.

Burke, a briskly efficient Aussie with a wry sense of humor, is something of an oddity in the sports science world. She essentially pioneered her position as head of sports nutrition at the AIS in 1990, a role that has grown to the point that she now leads a team of sixteen people. Over the years, she has helped bring scientific rigor to sports nutrition and has published hundreds of papers in peer-reviewed academic journals. And yet she is not an academic.

Her primary role at the AIS is to work "at the coalface," as she puts it, helping Australian athletes to bring home medals from international competitions like the Olympics. And she has learned that, whatever the peer-reviewed literature may say on any controversial topic, "it's important to listen to the athletes." Early in her career, she and her colleagues were convinced that you needed a relatively high dose of caffeine, taken well in advance of your race, to get a performance boost. But they couldn't figure out why cyclists stubbornly insisted on drinking flat cola late in multi-hour races. To prove the cyclists wrong, Burke and her colleagues designed a double-blinded, placebo-controlled test of low-dose caffeine during exercise—and discovered that it worked, an insight that has a lot to do with the current ubiquity of caffeine-spiked energy gels.

So, as LCHF continued to gain currency among endurance athletes, Burke decided it was worth returning to the topic for a more rigorous test of the Schwatka-style paradigm proposed by Phinney. The result was the Supernova mega-study, featuring a longer three-week period of fat adaptation and a much higher proportion of fat in the diet, as Phinney had prescribed. That's what brought Evan Dunfee and his fellow racewalkers to Canberra in late 2015—because if any athletes on the Olympic program stand to benefit from LCHF, it should be them. The men's 50-kilometer racewalk is among the longest events in the Olympics, with winning times just under four hours; also, the rules of sport forbid you from breaking into an all-out sprint, making the possible loss of high-end power less of a problem.

The Supernova results, which were published in 2017, confirmed that endurance athletes on a three-week high-fat diet became fat-burning machines to an extent few had imagined possible. By the end of a 25-kilometer time trial at their expected 50-kilometer race pace, the athletes were burning through 1.57 grams of fat per minute, which is two and a half times greater than the "normal" values seen in athletes eating a standard carbohydrate diet. That was the good news. The problem was that the fat-adapted athletes became less efficient, requiring more oxygen to sustain their race pace. This, it turns out, is a consequence of the cascade of metabolic reactions required to transform either fat or carbohydrate into ATP, the final form of fuel used for muscle contractions: the fat reactions require more oxygen molecules. If you're out for a leisurely stroll, that's no big deal, but if you're running (or walking) a race at a pace that leaves you out of breath, anything that forces you to consume *more* oxygen is a liability. As a result, it was no surprise that the LCHF athletes ended up performing worse than the high-carbohydrate athletes in the Supernova study's final and most important real-world test: a 10-kilometer racewalk.

That's bad news for would-be LCHF Olympians, but—as Burke acknowledges—it's *still* not the final nail in the coffin for the high-fat approach. After all, recreational ultra-endurance athletes may be more willing to accept an efficiency penalty in exchange for the freedom to refuel less frequently. The efficiency penalty may also be less pronounced at the slower paces sustainable in longer events like Ironman triathlons. And finally, there was the encouraging real-world performance of the athletes in the study in the weeks following their LCHF block: in addition to Dunfee's national 50-kilometer record, another walker from the study set an African record in the same race, and several others notched personal bests. At the Olympics later that summer, Dunfee earned minor celebrity status when he declined to appeal a ruling that left him in fourth place after the eventual bronze medalist, Japan's Hirooki Arai, was first disqualified for bumping Dunfee in the last kilometer of the race then subsequently reinstated. Dunfee left Rio without a medal, but with yet another national record, international acclaim for his sportsmanship, and lingering curiosity about the delayed benefits of the LCHF diet.

The upshot was that Burke reconvened an even larger group of race-walkers in Canberra in 2017 for Supernova 2, this time with a longer follow-up period to determine if a three-week LCHF block might deliver metabolic benefits that don't show up right away but kick in after the return to a high-carbohydrate diet. The results aren't yet available as I write this; but whatever happens, the surge of interest in LCHF means we'll soon know more than we did before about how different kinds of metabolic fuel affect the limits of endurance. "Nutrition is a cyclical science," Burke says. "You'd be surprised at how many 'new ideas' are simply old ideas reimagined. So there is always the chance that it's simply 'hula hoop season' again, and it will be a craze until it's not. But there's also a chance that new science will emerge."

For now, Burke is betting on a "periodized" approach to carbohydrate and fat during training—that is, carefully selecting certain workouts to perform with full carbohydrate reserves and others to do on empty. The goal isn't necessarily to boost fat usage in competition; instead, the carbohydrate-depleted workouts function as the nutritional equivalent of a weighted vest, forcing the body to work harder and triggering greater fitness gains in response. The problem with these bonk-prone depleted workouts is that they tend to be poor quality, which is why they need to be mixed with other workouts where you have enough carbohydrate to sustain high intensities. Burke and others published a pair of studies in 2016 using a protocol dubbed "sleep low," which involved a high-quality carbohydrate-fueled workout in the late afternoon, followed by a carbohydrate-free dinner; then, the next morning, a carbohydrate-depleted moderate workout before breakfast. Repeating this cycle just three times, for a total of six days, produced a 3 percent improvement in 20-kilometer cycling times.

Such protocols (and even the word *protocol* itself) make the idea of deliberately depleted training seem highly regimented and scientific. But as Burke herself points out, athletes in many sports have stumbled into similar patterns over the years, either by design or from necessity. Cycling legend Miguel Indurain is rumored to have made five-hour rides on an empty stomach a staple of his training in the 1990s; Kenyan runners, despite their heavy reliance on carbohydrates, often start out in such poverty that they frequently train hungry. And mountain climbers, too, have learned to train in ways that ramp up fat-burning without sacrificing their carbohydrate capacity during arduous multiday expeditions—an approach to metabolic flexibility forged in an environment where the consequences of "bonking" can be fatal.

In June 2000, the alpinists Steve House, Mark Twight, and Scott Backes set out to climb the South Face of Denali, the highest peak in North

America, via an obscure and challenging route known as the Slovak Direct. The first (and eponymous) ascent of this route, in 1986, took eleven days and required a thousand feet of fixed rope bolted into the rock and ice along the route. The second ascent took seven days. Now, for the third ascent, House and his climbing partners were bringing no tent, no sleeping bags, and a minimum of rope. They planned to climb the entire route in a single push.

In some ways, mountaineering is an ideal test bed for experimenting with energy limits. In alpine-style ascents, you have to carry everything you plan to eat—no small inconvenience when you're ascending pitch after pitch of vertical ice walls. And the typical intensity required during climbing, which is around 65 to 75 percent of your aerobic maximum, is ideal for relying on your copious fat stores. "The food bag in your pack is heavy, yet we already carry lots of energy with us all the time," House and his coach, Scott Johnston, explain in *Training for the New Alpinism: A Manual for the Climber as Athlete.* "The trick is to train your body and eat strategically so that you burn lots of this energy source and need less food." That means making sure you get enough fat as part of a balanced training diet (for House, that meant upping the fat content in his diet from 5 percent to 30 percent); doing plenty of moderate-intensity endurance training; and perhaps even doing multi-hour fasted training sessions first thing in the morning, an approach House experimented with and found useful.

Those were the fixes Johnson and House prescribed to the prominent climber and mountain guide Adrian Ballinger, who enlisted their coaching services following a failed attempt to summit Everest without supplemental oxygen in 2016. Lab testing at UC Davis's sports performance lab showed that Ballinger's metabolism shifted from burning predominantly fat to predominantly carbohydrate at a relatively low heart rate of 115 beats per minute. In the "death zone" near the summit of Everest, where appetite is suppressed and digestion and other bodily functions begin to shut down, this carbohydrate dependence left him starved of energy, shivering uncontrollably, with hands so numb that he could no longer work the carabiners that protected him. Wisely, he turned back two hours from the summit.

To help Ballinger tap into his fat stores more effectively, Johnston told him to add fasted endurance workouts to his training and shift to a higher-fat diet. The changes were initially challenging: Ballinger's usual twelve mile runs turned into seven miles slogs taking the same amount of time. But before long, he was going out for five-hour workouts without needing to eat anything. A return visit to the lab four months later confirmed that his fat-carbohydrate crossover point had moved from 115 to 141 beats per minute, allowing him to rely more on fat during moderate-intensity ascents and preserve his precious carbohydrate stores for when they were really needed. In the spring of 2017, Ballinger and his climbing partner Cory Richards returned to Everest, with Johnston and House monitoring their uploaded heart rate data from afar. On the 12-mile climb to Advance Base Camp, higher than the highest point in North America, Ballinger's heart rate was below 120; two days later, climbing to the North Col, it stayed below 125. The difference from the previous year was dramatic, and on May 27, Ballinger joined the very short list, started less than four decades earlier by Messner and Habeler, of those who have stood on the roof of the world powered by their lungs alone.

It would be a mistake, though, to consider this feat a triumph of fat and nothing else. You train to burn fat, House says, but you race on carbs. Once you're in the mountains, in other words, you try, as Louise Burke counsels, to maximize every metabolic pathway you've got by hitting the carbohydrates as hard as you can. On Slovak Direct, in 2000, House and his partners packed 144 energy gels—pure carbohydrate—based on the assumption that each person would eat one gel per hour for forty-eight hours and nothing else. With this approach, balancing the need for external carbs with the benefits of a light pack and the baseline energy from their fat stores, they figured they would be able make it to the top—just barely—before running out of fuel.

After twenty-four hours of climbing, House, Twight, and Backes had passed the point of no return: they no longer had enough anchors to descend via the route they had climbed. As the hours wore on, they struggled with sleep deprivation, numbing cold, and simple physical exhaustion. Alternating between rock and ice, they had to stop twice to file their dulled climbing tools. After forty-eight hours they ran out of fuel for the two stoves they had brought to melt water. Thanks to effort- and altitude-induced nausea, they fell behind on their gel-eating schedule. Their energy levels began to run dangerously low. The warning signs grew louder: "The cramps were fierce and the aural hallucinations memorable," Twight later recalled.

Once again, in other words, the limits facing House and his companions as they clung to the icy mountainside were, quite literally, echoing in their heads. As with all the other limiters we've discussed in the past six chapters, the ultimate physical crisis—in this case, muscles that cease to contract due to a lack of fuel—is preceded by a steadily escalating series of alarms. The low-fuel alarms are particularly loud and insistent, and provide some of the most compelling evidence of involuntary anticipatory regulation: the boost derived from swishing and spitting a sports drink; the impaired efficiency of a muscle fiber whose fuel stores are still half-full. But they can still be ignored for a time. Most American climbers, Twight argues, "are scared to be hungry, or they wouldn't carry so much damn food."

House, Twight, and Backes tempted their own limits; in a mental fog, they briefly got lost trying to skirt a huge serac that dominates Denali's South Face. But they eventually found a line of climbable mixed terrain between the serac and the steepest section of rock, and got back on track. Finally, after sixty hours of nonstop climbing, exhausted, starving, dehydrated, and sleep-deprived, they made it to the top. Then, like a marathoner who staggers through the finish line and keeps jogging, they carried on—because they still had to get back down.

Two Hours

March 6, 2017

A disaster is unfolding in slow motion before us. Since the race-track was built in 1922, Italy's Autodromo Nazionale Monza—the so-called Temple of Speed—has echoed with the high-octane roar of epic races, hosted countless speed records (at 231.523 mph, which Colombian driver Juan Pablo Montoya reached in the 2005 Italian Grand Prix, a marathon would take less than seven minutes), and mourned the deaths of more than fifty drivers and forty spectators, mostly in the freewheeling early days of motorsport. On this bright, early March day in northern Italy, though, the problem is the pacers.

Kipchoge, Tadese, and Desisa are here to run a half-marathon dress rehearsal for their attempt at the full distance, which is now slated for early May. While Nike announced its Breaking2 project to the world back in December, it has chosen to keep most of the details secret, which has generated curiosity and resentment in roughly equal pro-portions. With the shoes and the drafting plan under wraps, most observers have assumed either that Nike is simply drumming up pub-licity by attacking an impossible goal, or that they're planning to cheat outrageously with a downhill course or wheeled shoes or some other gimmick. The details of the attempt were finally released at a press conference earlier this morning. Now, with the whole running world watching closely, Nike's scientific team will get a chance to see how all the tweaks and nudges and harebrained schemes they've been sweat-ing over in the lab play out in the real world.

A few hours before the start, Brad Wilkins, Nike's director of Next Generation Research, gives me a quick tour of the course. The 1.5-mile

"Junior Course" is almost perfectly flat, with a total rise and fall of just 18 feet per loop. Monza is located only 600 feet above sea level, which means the runners will get a full lungful of oxygen with each breath—it's low enough to avoid the problems I experienced at 1,900 feet in Canberra (see page 133). Striding down the course's majestic finishing straight, Wilkins points out the pancake-flat timing mats that will wirelessly beam real-time pace feedback every 400 meters (they will be twice as frequent at the final event), and the two weather stations his team has installed to gather track-level data on temperature, humidity, and wind speed. The temperature in early May should be in the low 50s, cool enough to avoid overheating and minimize the risk of dehydration. Today's wind, he acknowledges, is bad—bad enough to merit postponing the attempt if this were the real thing, which is why the final event will take place during a three-day "launch window" rather than on a predetermined date. "And as a physiologist," he deadpans, glancing up at a shimmering azure sky dotted with a few puffs of white cloud, "another thing I don't like is the sun. Too much radiant heat."

Finally, with the bleat of an asthmatic-sounding airhorn, the runners set off, following a sleek (and exhaust-free) black Tesla pace car with a Formula One test driver at the wheel. The first six pacemakers quickly coalesce into an arrowhead formation in rows of one, two, and three, a configuration that has been optimized in wind-tunnel testing and in computational fluid dynamics simulations run by an aerodynamics whiz in New Hampshire. It's an impressive sight—but it doesn't last. One pacemaker soon pulls up lame, and another can't hold the pace. Even after replacements are swapped in, the runners struggle to maintain their tightly choreographed positioning while running so uncomfortably close to one another at such a fast pace. The arrowhead soon dissolves into more of a loose amoeba formation, leaving Kipchoge and his teammates partly exposed.

Worse, before they even reach halfway, Desisa starts to drift off the back. Wilkins has been adamant that the half-marathon is a purely logistical exercise; the athletes, after all, are in the midst of heavy training, with Desisa reportedly exceeding two hundred miles a week. "We're not trying to test the athletes' fitness," he insists. "We're testing ourselves." Still, as Desisa's deficit stretches from feet to yards to dozens of yards, the crew at the finish exchange worried glances. Despite all the science, the best athletes in the world, the millions of dollars, it's clear that failure *is* an option.

For the first time in my career, I've been getting hate mail—accusations that I'm a Nike shill, that through my coverage of the project I'm complicit in defiling the purity of running and turning the sport into a novelty sideshow. Though I'm surprised by the vehemence, I understand where it's coming from. Running's simplicity is its defining characteristic; it's why so many champions come from the poorest regions of the world, and why the International Association of Athletics Federations, the sport's governing body, has 214 affiliated countries and territories—more than the United Nations. And the marathon itself has its own rich history, which sits uneasily with top-secret shoes, arrowhead drafting formations, and rule-flouting exhibitions planned by PR-savvy mega-corporations.

It's not, the critics point out, like the good old days when Roger Bannister broke the four-minute mile while training on his lunch break from his medical studies. This is undoubtedly true in some respects—but there are a surprising number of parallels between the sub-two and sub-four chases. For one thing, Bannister's feat was accomplished in a series of carefully orchestrated time trials, rather than in head-to-head competition with John Landy or other sub-four aspirants. In 1953, Bannister took part in a special exhibition during a high school meet in which he was paced for two and a half laps by one runner, after which his Oxford teammate Chris Brasher, who had allowed himself to be lapped while jogging, paced him for the rest of the race. Bannister's time of 4:02.0 wasn't recognized as a British record, because it violated exactly the same pacing rules as Nike's Breaking2 race—but the run served its purpose. "[O]nly two painful seconds now separated me from the four-minute mile," he later explained, "and I was certain I could cut down the time."

Nike's scientists advance basically the same argument: if Kipchoge or one of his teammates succeeds in breaking two hours under the artificial conditions in Monza, it will pave the way for someone else to do it in a regular big-city race. The mind, in other words, frames the outer limits of what we believe is humanly possible.

The debate brings to mind the arguments about supplemental oxygen on Mount Everest. When the first British expeditions attacked the mountain in the 1920s, the technology was still in its infancy, but some expedition members felt its use was unsporting and would tarnish their intended accomplishment. In the end, when Edmund Hillary and Tenzing Norgay finally scaled the mountain in 1953, they did use oxygen. Another twenty-five years passed before Messner and Habeler's oxygen-free first ascent. Would their feat have been possible without the route-finding and trail-blazing of the aided climbers who went before them? "Never" is a long time, but I suspect the mountain would still be unclimbed to this day.

The shoes add yet another wrinkle. On the day of the half-marathon, the *New York Times* publishes a grainy CT scan of a prototype, sent in by Yannis Pitsiladis, who heads a rival sub-two initiative, in which the carbon-fiber plate looks like a hidden knife revealed by airport security. The plate, the *Times* claims, is "meant to act as a kind of slingshot, or catapult, to propel runners forward." Are such shoes, with their reported 4 percent efficiency boost, really fair?

In a way, running is facing the same dilemma that confronted cycling's governing body in the 1990s when they decided to "freeze" the technology permissible for the Hour record, and that faced swimming when they decided to ban polyurethane "fast suits" in 2010. Technology evolves, but when it evolves so quickly that it effectively picks winners, that's a problem. The top three finishers in the men's Olympic marathon in 2016, it turns out, were wearing disguised prototypes of the new shoe, which Nike has dubbed the Vaporfly. So was the women's winner; so were the men's winners of the 2016 London, Chicago,

Berlin, and New York marathons. If we're interested in human limits, what does a sub-two-hour marathon truly tell us if all it takes is a 2:03 runner wearing supershoes?

All these questions are lurking below the surface as I watch Kipchoge power around the track for his final lap, while the late afternoon sun sinks behind the cavernously empty grandstands. Tadese, too, has fallen behind, but Kipchoge still has a light, almost effortless bounce to his stride. He crosses the finish line in a hard-to-fathom time of 59:19 and saunters over to a nearby scale, where Andrew Jones is waiting to weigh him in order to calculate his sweat losses. Tadese follows in 59:42, faster than Ryan Hall's American record of 59:43. He could have gone faster, he later explains, but chose to stick instead to the pre-race plan of aiming for 60 minutes. Desisa, downcast but determined to finish, notches a 1:02:56.

After cooling down and getting their sweats on, the runners good-naturedly field questions from the scrum of journalists. In addition to the usual sports reporters, there are representatives from design magazines, health shows, fashion blogs. Desisa mentions a nagging injury; Kipchoge volleys a series of oddball questions (Did you have any meals? "Well, I had lunch." But during the race, did you have any meals? "No, no meals during the race." Is that a problem? Would you normally have a meal during a marathon? "No, you don't need any meals during a marathon.") before I ask the big one: How hard did he have to push to run 59:19? Was it 95 percent effort? Ninety-eight percent? One hundred? He grins. "Sixty percent," he says. "It was part of my training."

The next day dawns crisp, sunny, and without a breath of wind—as if to prove Wilkins's point about the benefits of a three-day launch window. It's debriefing time for the science and operations teams. The shoe guys take close-up photographs of the race-worn prototypes, looking for telltale wrinkles in the foam or wear patterns on the sole that suggest needed tweaks. Desisa, chastened, agrees to switch from his familiar split-shorts, which he had chosen to wear at the last min-ute, to the new high-tech half-tights. And the physiologists begin to sift through data collected by core-temperature pills that the runners swallowed before the race, as well as from taped-on muscle oxygen and skin-temperature sensors, to get a sense of whether they could have maintained the pace for twice as long. An encouraging sign: Kip-choge's core temperature has barely budged from start to finish, with no signs of incipient overheating. "One thing that was awesome about today," says Wilkins, who's itching to start the analysis, "is that no-body has data on a 59:19 half-marathon. We have that now. So you put those into the models—we could break the models!"

As impressive as Kipchoge's run is, though, it's not unprecedented. Thirty-three men have run faster than 59:19; none of them has come within shouting distance of a two-hour marathon. His claim that his effort was just "sixty percent" might be bravado; it might be nervous humor. But by May 6, 2017, the tentative date of the Breaking2 run (chosen because it's the anniversary of Bannister's sub-four), the truth will out.

In interviews over the weeks that follow, Kipchoge returns again and again to the theme of belief. "The verdict was that I'm ready to attempt the unknown through faith by believing in myself," he tells a Kenyan reporter who asks about the results of all the physiological testing he underwent at Nike headquarters in Oregon. "The difference only is thinking," he tells another reporter: "You think it's impossible, I think it's possible."

But is it realistic for an Olympic champion who has been at the top of his game for over a decade to push back his brain's limit settings even further? And if so, how?

Part III

LIMIT BREAKERS

CHAPTER 11

Training the Brain

In the opening chapters of this book, I set up a tidy choice between the "human machine" view of endurance, in which your limits are reached when, say, your muscles can't get enough oxygen or your fuel tank is empty, and the "it's all in your head" view, in which failure is either a choice or an act of self-protection. Over the six preceding chapters, we've tried to see which of those worldviews best fits the facts in the face of various extreme challenges. And the answer, I have to confess, isn't as obvious as I thought it would be when I first started working on this book.

Think back to Tim Noakes's observation about the second-place Olympic marathoner jogging around the track waving his country's flag. "Do you notice he's not dead?" he asked. "It means he could have run faster." But in some situations—fortunately rare—people *do* die while trying to stretch the limits of their endurance: Henry Worsley skiing to exhaustion in Antarctica; Max Gilpin running until his cells sizzled in the heat; freedivers who don't make it back to the surface before the lights go out. In each of these cases, you could argue that the circumstances are unusual or that some external factor, like an infection, intervened. But the fact remains that humans do sometimes reach limits that are concrete and immutable. Sometimes, no matter who is trapped under the wheels, you can't lift the car.

Having accepted that somewhat deflating reality, it's worth reflecting on a common thread that runs through those six chapters. How you reach the ultimate endpoint at which you beg for mercy or fall off the treadmill depends very much on the particular circumstances—

whether you're starved of oxygen on an alpine summit, parched and roasting in the desert, or trying to coax one more step from fuel-depleted muscles. But in each case, long before you reach that point of extremity, you'll be feeling the effects. At first you might not notice the subtle change, but gradually the effort required to sustain your pace will grow until you become conscious that you won't be able to continue forever—that the unforgiving minute must eventually end. At this point, your core temperature is still within the normal range, your muscles still have all the fuel and oxygen they need, and the metabolic by-products of exercise haven't yet accumulated to a level that interferes with your forward progress. Only your brain knows that trouble is coming. But the clock is still ticking.

Samuele Marcora would argue that this growing sense of effort is all that matters—that we pace ourselves to keep the effort manageable, and quit when it gets higher than we're willing to tolerate. In contrast, Noakes, drawing on the work of collaborators such as Alan St. Clair Gibson, sees the sense of effort as a conscious manifestation of hard-wired neural circuitry that kicks in to hold us back from the precipice. One of Marcora's most powerful arguments is the simplicity of his theory: he himself draws the comparison to the pursuit, in physics, of a single Grand Unified Theory that can explain the whole universe. But there's another physics analogy that this debate reminds me of: the dispute between various interpretations of quantum mechanics (Copenhagen, many-worlds, De Broglie-Bohm) that all converge on the same set of equations and predictions. They're different ways of thinking about the same thing.

In 2009, one of Noakes's former students, Ross Tucker, published a paper in the *British Journal of Sports Medicine* on the "anticipatory regulation of performance," in which he tried to explain how, exactly, the brain knows in advance to slow you down before catastrophe strikes. What single mechanism integrates information about body temperature, oxygen levels, and fuel storage, and also responds to more subtle indicators like your mood and how much you slept last night? The answer, Tucker suggested, was Borg's rating of perceived exertion, or RPE, which he described as "the conscious/verbal manifestation of the integration of these psychological and physiological cues." Moreover, this effort rating climbs gradually as body temperature increases or carbohydrate stores decrease: it doesn't just wait for the catastrophe; it anticipates it.

Pacing, in Tucker's formulation, is the process of comparing the effort you feel at any given point in a race to the effort you expect at that stage—an internal template that you develop and fine-tune from experience. If the start of a race feels like a 10 out of 20 effort on the Borg scale, and you expect to hit 20 by the end, then halfway through the race the effort should feel like a 15. If, instead, you're at 16 halfway through the race, you'll feel a powerful urge to slow down—even though you're still far from the max of 20. In this picture, my struggles when I moved up from 1,500-meter to 5,000-meter races (as described in Chapter 3) were the result of an ill-formed pacing template. In the fourth kilometer of each race, when I felt unable to maintain my pace, it was because of a mismatch between anticipated and actual effort, not because I was hitting a physical limit. That's why, in the final laps where I *expected* effort to be near-maximal, I was suddenly able to speed up again.

Is this really an explanation of how endurance is regulated, or is it simply a description of how it feels? This is where the debate gets heated. No one actually calculates and consciously verbalizes Borg ratings during a race; instead, this process takes place somewhere under the hood. Where Marcora disagrees with Tucker and Noakes is in the extent to which such decisions and computations take place consciously and voluntarily versus unconsciously and automatically. They also disagree about the role of feedback from throughout the body to the brain in generating the sensation of effort: Marcora believes such feedback contributes to feelings of pain and discomfort but not effort, which is instead dictated by the brain's *outgoing* signals to the muscles. And lurking uncomfortably in the background of their debates is the question of who gets the credit for developing these ideas. But where they agree is on the centrality of effort. How hard it feels dictates, in a true and literal sense and with greater accuracy than any physiological measurement yet devised, how long you can sustain it.

As in the famous Emo Phillips joke about the schism between the Northern Conservative Baptist Great Lakes Region Council of 1879 and the Northern Conservative Baptist Great Lakes Region Council of 1912, the bitterest debates often seem to arise where the substantive differences are smallest. There are, to be sure, many questions that remain to be answered about the brain's role in endurance. But on the central question, in my view, Marcora, Tucker, and Noakes are now saying essentially the same thing. Effort is what matters.

Once you accept that conclusion, an inevitable question looms: how do you train effort? The standard answer, and still the best one, is that you train your body. If you want running at 5:00-mile pace to feel easier, you should head out the door and run at 5:00-mile pace—a lot. Over time, your heart will get stronger, your muscles will grow more energy-producing mitochondria, and you'll sprout new capillaries to distribute oxygen-rich blood. These changes will allow you to sustain 5:00 pace with less physiological strain, and they'll also attenuate the distress signals that your muscles and heart send back to the brain. The pace will *feel* easier, so you'll be able to sustain it for longer. Explaining the effects of training by talking about effort rather than, say, VO_2max is a provocative shift in perspective, but it doesn't really tell us anything new about how to train.

There is one important difference, though. Effort is no longer just a by-product of the physiological strain that causes you to slow down or stop; in the effort-centered view, as the diagram on page 59 illustrates, effort is what *causes* you to slow down or stop. So anything that moves the "effort dial" in your head up or down will affect your endurance, even if it has no effect on your muscles or heart or VO_2max. That was the claim that caught my attention during Samuele Marcora's conference presentation in Australia in 2010, and it represents his most original and significant insight. It's why he has conducted military-funded studies of caffeine gum, which alters perception of effort by blocking the buildup of fatigue-related brain chemicals. It's why he has shown that subliminal images of effort-related words, or even smiling or frowning faces, can alter the perception of effort and thus increase or decrease endurance. And it's why he came up with the idea of "brain endurance training."

On my first day at the University of Kent's picturesque campus in the British seaside town of Chatham, I threw up in the bushes. Twice. I had convinced my editors at *Runner's World* to send me to Marcora's lab to learn more about his brain-training theories, so that I could try them out myself while preparing for my first marathon. Shortly before my visit, Marcora's colleague Alexis Mauger had published a highly controversial study using a new effort-based protocol to measure VO_2max. Instead of putting subjects through a "brainless" test where the speed increases in set increments, Mauger's subjects ran or cycled at steadily increasing levels of self-determined effort. The results, which remain highly contentious, showed that subjects reached higher VO_2max values in the effort-based test than in the traditional test—an impossible paradox if you believe that VO_2max represents a physical ceiling on oxygen consumption.

Mauger, a laid-back senior lecturer in jeans and flip-flops, offered to run me through the new test so I could compare it to my previous experiences with the standard test. He fitted a mask over my mouth and tied me into a safety harness dangling from the roof. "Just in case," he said, a little too cheerfully. "That last stage can be pretty tough." The biggest adjustment was that, in order to maintain a relatively constant effort (12 out of 20 for the first stage, for example), I had to start out quickly and then gradually reduce the pace during each two-minute stage as my legs fatigued. For the last stage, which called for two minutes at an all-out effort of 20, I had to start out as if I were sprinting a 100-meter dash and then gradually decrease the treadmill speed just enough to avoid being thrown off the back as I tired. Balancing on the edge of that red line was, quite literally, gut-churningly hard. Fortunately, I made it back out to the parking lot before hurling.

Mauger's study was copublished in the *British Journal of Sports Medicine* alongside another study, from Noakes's group in Cape Town, that also used a novel protocol to produce higher-than-"max" VO$_2$max values. That study, which was led by Noakes's student Fernando Beltrami, used a similar "reverse" protocol that started fast and gradually slowed down just enough to enable the subjects to stay on the treadmill as they tired. One of the curious details of Beltrami's study was that, when the subjects returned to the lab for a follow-up test using the conventional accelerating VO$_2$max protocol, their values stayed at the new, higher value. To Beltrami, who also coaches runners, this suggests that the mere fact of having attained the higher level of oxygen consumption somehow adjusts the brain's settings. He has since been experimenting with using the reverse VO$_2$max protocol as a training tool, for example incorporating it into the preparations of an athlete training for a 100-kilometer race in Patagonia.

This idea of adjusting the brain's settings evokes a long-standing debate: who has to work harder, a 2:30 marathoner or a 3:30 marathoner? One standard (if deliberately provocative) answer is that the 3:30 marathoner has a harder task, because she has to spend an extra hour pushing her limits. But I've always thought that a better proxy for who works harder (on average, of course) is cumulative years and volume of training, not finishing time. The process of training expands the capabilities of the muscles and heart, sure, but it also recalibrates the brain's horizons. As we saw in Chapter 5, trained ultra-runners have a higher pain tolerance than nonathletes, and even over the course of a single year the pain tolerance of athletes waxes and wanes with training cycles. In this sense, all training is brain training, even if it doesn't specifically target the brain.

At the first beeping of my watch alarm, I spring out of bed, pull on my running shorts and trainers, slather on sunscreen, and sit down at my computer. It's 7 A.M. on a Sunday in mid-May, several months after my visit to Kent and just two weeks before the start of my first marathon, and time for my final big test. On the screen, an empty road disappears into a blue sky dotted with drifting clouds, rendered in simple 1980s-video-game graphics. With a sigh, I empty my mind and click a blue button marked START, bracing myself for the drudgery ahead. Shapes begin flashing on the screen, sometimes to the left of the road and sometimes to the right. When it's a triangle, I hit a button corresponding to the side of the screen it's on as quickly as possible, usually within a few hundred milliseconds. When it's a circle, I do nothing. If I fail to respond within two seconds, or respond when I shouldn't, the screen flashes red and the computer buzzes angrily.

And that's it. For the next sixty minutes, my sole task is to keep my brain locked on this excruciatingly dull parade of shapes. They flash by rapidly, leaving no time to daydream, check the clock, or even glance out the window. Still, thoughts occasionally intrude. I find myself wondering how hot it is outside, and whether I should have started earlier—then *bam,* the screen buzzes red. The longer I go, the more frequent my mistakes become. When the hour is finally up, I have that cotton-headed feeling of total mental exhaustion that's usually the cue to flop down in front of the TV for a few hours. Instead, I down a glass of water, step outside into the blinding sunshine, and start running.

I lope through two miles, then gradually squeeze the pace down. I have a fifteen-mile progression run planned, with the last six at marathon race pace. My legs feel fine, but there's a persistent mismatch between the effort I'm feeling and the splits on my watch—the pace feels tougher than it should, and I have to concentrate to sustain it. Once again, I force my brain to zero in on a monotonous task: keeping my legs moving and hitting my goal splits, instead of watching shapes on a screen. As far as my brain is concerned, the effort feels more like the last fifteen miles of a marathon than the first fifteen—which means the plan is working.

While all training may be brain training, my visit to Marcora's lab introduced me to techniques that zero in on the specific aspects of brain function that limit endurance. As we saw in Chapter 4, he and others have identified a cognitive trait called response inhibition, which involves overriding your initial instinct, as a key. A psychologist at the University of Portsmouth in Britain, Chris Wagstaff, offered a particularly graphic illustration of its importance for athletes. He asked cyclists to watch a three-minute video showing "an Asian woman causing herself to throw up and who subsequently eats her own vomit." Some of the volunteers were instructed to suppress any emotions and keep a poker face while watching, while others weren't given any instructions. In a subsequent 10-kilometer time trial, those who had kept a poker face cycled more slowly right from the start, and experienced higher perceived effort. After one kilometer, the poker-face group reported an average effort rating of almost 15 out of 20, compared to 12 in the control group, despite going slower. That's a huge difference.

How do you improve your response inhibition? By inhibiting your responses, over and over, in a systematic way. Marcora's mental fatigue studies use a set of standard cognitive tasks that can be tailored to tax different aspects of cognitive control, including response inhibition. After my adventures with Mauger's VO_2max test, Marcora introduced me to Walter Staiano, his postdoctoral research associate, who ushered me into a carpeted room with a big poster of Usain Bolt on the wall and an exercise bike surrounded by computer screens and jumbled cables and wires. After affixing electrodes to my bald pate to monitor my brain activity, he parked me on the bike and told me to follow the instructions on the screen while pedaling at a comfortable pace. My task: when five arrows flashed onto the pixelated road-and-sky backdrop of the screen, I was to ignore four of them and press a key indicating which direction the middle arrow was pointing. I did a double take as I read the instructions.

"That's *it*?" I asked, recalling Marcora's warnings about how horrible these studies were.

"That's it," Staiano replied. "You can start whenever you're ready."

The task was laughably easy—at first. And as the seconds dragged by and arrows kept flashing, it didn't get any harder. But I soon developed a very strong desire to do something else. Anything else. My mind wandered: I started thinking about the questions I wanted to ask Marcora, and whether I'd have time to go back to my hotel before lunch. Suddenly a buzzer sounded and the screen flashed red: I'd pressed the wrong button. Chastened, I refocused on the screen. After a while, I figured I must have done enough of that particular task, so I suggested that we move on to the next one. I asked Staiano how long I'd lasted. "Five minutes." Staiano grinned. "In the mental fatigue studies, they do ninety minutes." Suddenly, I understood why Marcora's subjects hated him.

Funded by the British military's Centre for Defence Enterprise, Marcora has spent the last few years experimenting with various brain endurance training protocols—three or five days a week, thirty to sixty minutes per session, sitting at a computer or riding on a stationary bike. In addition to the flashing arrows, he has also tried other cognitive tasks involving shapes and letters. So to aid my preparations for that spring's Ottawa Marathon, he helped me devise a twelve-week routine, five days a week, rotating through three different cognitive tasks (arrows, shapes, letters), starting with extremely modest sessions of fifteen minutes and progressing, if all went well, to an hour and a half. By triggering the flood of neurotransmitters associated with mental fatigue and, in particular, response inhibition over and over, we hoped that my brain would adapt to the insult—and that my resistance to mental fatigue would translate into an ability to sustain a slightly faster pace at the same effort.

I should pause here to acknowledge the obvious: I have no way of assessing whether the mental training actually helped my marathon.

That's actually part of the reason I chose the marathon, a distance I had never run before, as a test—to avoid misleading comparisons with previous races. Rather than a "study," I viewed my experiment as a chance to find out what brain endurance training *felt* like. Would it be tolerable? Enjoyable? Impossible? To that end, when I returned home and started training for the race, I tried to suppress my skepticism and follow the program.

It wasn't easy. Initially, I rotated through the three different training tasks in five-minute blocks, figuring variety would help stave off boredom. But when I emailed Marcora to double-check this approach, he had bad news: "Being boring is an important characteristic for inducing mental fatigue and, therefore, a brain training effect," he replied. "Just do a longer session of one test at a time." After a few weeks, I'd progressed to thirty-minute brain sessions. Sometimes, following Marcora's advice, I ran immediately after, to practice running while mentally fatigued. The result was strikingly familiar: it felt like heading out for a run immediately after a stressful work or travel day (which is why one of Marcora's practical tips for incorporating brain training into your routine is to occasionally hit the gym after a long workday, rather than always training when you're mentally fresh). It wasn't so much that I couldn't run faster—it just felt harder than usual in a way that was difficult to pin down. I'd check my pace partway through a run, realize that I needed to speed up, but somehow be unable to summon the willpower to make it happen.

Ten weeks before the race, I tested my fitness in a half-marathon. I was satisfied with my time of 1:15, but not with the distribution of my effort. My first and last 5K segments were the fastest, while the middle segments were the slowest—a failure of concentration reminiscent of my struggles with 5,000-meter races during my track-running heyday. I scheduled my next test race four weeks later, and in the meantime pushed my computer sessions to 60 and then 80 minutes. In that next half-marathon, I managed just under 1:13, and my splits revealed good news: I'd managed to keep pushing at a steady pace through the middle miles, and this time my last few miles were the slowest. In an odd way, this late-race fade was exactly what I'd been striving for. Maybe, just maybe, the brain training was kicking in.

On race day in Ottawa, I hit the halfway point in 1:18:25, right on pace for my goal time of 2:37 (a challenging but relatively sensible target given my half-marathon times). My breathing was smooth, my legs felt good, and my mind was acutely tuned to my pace. Of course, everyone feels that way halfway through a marathon—I knew the real test was still to come. I had planned some additional tricks to help manipulate my effort during the second half of the race. To harness the brain-fooling effects of carbohydrate in the mouth, I was swishing and spitting sports drink at every opportunity. And based on Marcora's research linking facial expression to perceived effort, I'd positioned friends and family at regular intervals along the course with instructions to make me smile.

At one point, I rounded a corner and spotted my friend Shannon on the roadside holding a giant yellow sign that read: REMEMBER WHEN I BROUGHT YOU BURMESE FOOD AND THEN ATE IT? She'd once made an epic ten-hour drive back from Washington, D.C., (where I had previously spent a few years working) with an order of my favorite dish from my favorite restaurant on ice as a surprise, and then, after a friend mistakenly told her that I was out of town, slurped down the last bite just as I returned her call. Her husband, Geoff, stood beside her with an equally enormous sign that read simply, SHE'S SORRY! I spat out a mouthful of Powerade in a graceful electric-blue arc and broke into a grin.

Soon I was steadily passing other runners. It's not that I sped up; everyone else was just slowing down. In fact, I was a metronome, nailing each split to within a few seconds, with mental focus to spare. By the time I hit 30K in 1:51:35, still a few ticks under 2:37 pace, I was riding the high of a plan that seemed to be coming together perfectly. There was just one discordant note: my quads were starting to feel sore. Most of my training had been on hilly dirt trails, and my legs weren't used to the repetitive pounding of flat asphalt roads.

My wife, mother, and father had mapped out a series of cheering spots to sustain me during the crucial last 10K of the race. Each time I spotted one of them holding a sign or wearing a silly hat while scream-ing encouragement, I had more difficulty twisting my facial muscles in a smile. I thought back to what Marcora had told me about the dif-ference between effort and pain. We often think of races as "painful," but physical pain is completely distinct from the sense of effort—the struggle to keep going against a mounting desire to stop—that usually limits race speed. What I now felt in my quads was pain resulting from physical damage to the muscle fibers in my legs, an electric stab-bing sensation that my hours of clicking at the computer had done nothing to prepare me for—and it was rapidly approaching intolera-ble. I clicked a button on my watch as I passed the 35K mark. I was still on 2:38 pace, but the wheels were about to come off.

Over the last four miles, I had the surreal sensation that the race was running backward, as people I had passed during the middle miles started to pass me back. Even stranger, as the pain in my quads intensified, my overall sense of effort decreased—my breathing and heart rate slowed because my legs simply could no longer move fast enough to keep them elevated. I was reduced to a jog, frustrated but powerless to accelerate. I stopped checking splits and recalculating my finish time, because it was going to take all my mental strength to make it to the finish without walking.

After the race, I had the awkward task of writing a magazine article about my experience. After hobbling across the finish line in an unde-niably disappointing 2:44:48, what could I possibly say about whether brain endurance training really worked? When I contacted Marcora for a post-race debrief, what I most wanted to know was whether I could really blame my late-race fade on pain, rather than on a fail-ure of brain endurance. "Of course!" he said. "You had muscle pain which was so intense as to limit your performance." I could no more "run through" the damaged muscle fibers in my legs than I could run through a broken ankle, he explained. In most cases, exercise only generates moderate levels of muscle pain and is limited by extreme levels of effort. But sometimes, as I'd discovered, it's the other way around.

In the end, I did gain some insights from the experience. For one thing, brain endurance training is mind-numbingly boring; for another, it's incredibly time-consuming. For anyone whose athletic pursuits have to fit around family and job obligations, making time for marathon training is already tough enough. Adding in another hour or more a day is a big ask, especially when the benefits remain unproven. That's why Marcora's most recent studies have used a combined protocol where subjects do physical and mental training at the same time. In 2015, Staiano and Marcora presented recently declassified results from a military-funded study of thirty-five volunteers who had trained three times a week for an hour at a time on stationary bikes. Half of the volunteers did brain training while cycling, using the flashing-letters test that I had tried. After twelve weeks, the physical-training-only group had improved their time to exhaustion by 42 percent; in comparison the physical-plus-brain-training group had improved by a whopping 126 percent. This hybrid protocol is more time-efficient and less boring than the brain-training-only protocol I followed—and with effects that large, I suspect lots of people would be willing to endure a little boredom.

That's not to say brain endurance training is ready for prime time. The whole field of brain training, particularly as a tool to ward off cognitive decline, has been mired in controversy in recent years. It's now a billion-dollar industry, but a 2016 analysis of virtually every brain-training study ever published concluded that there is little evidence for "transferability"—that is, training yourself to click buttons in response to flashing letters or shapes doesn't necessarily translate into, say, remembering phone numbers or acing exams. Can it transfer to running a faster marathon? We should reserve judgment until those experiments have been completed and then confirmed by multiple researchers from different laboratories.

There's another important caveat, which is that Marcora's most impressive results are seen in previously untrained volunteers—a group that is primed to improve under almost any circumstances. But is the same true for athletes who are already engaged in the mentally demanding task of *physical* endurance training? Perhaps hours of focus during long bike rides or demanding trail runs hone your mental fitness to the point of diminishing returns. That's a possibility Marcora is well aware of, and he is currently planning brain training studies with elite athletes. And it's why he collaborated with researchers at the Australian Institute of Sport on the study of elite cyclists described on page 68—because one way to figure out how to make our brains better is to look at the brains of people who are *already* elite performers.

Entering the final length in the 200-meter freestyle final at the 2008 Beijing Olympics, swimmer Sara Isaković tucked into her flip turn, uncoiled her legs, and felt . . . nothing. Instead of exploding off the wall, the twenty-year-old Slovenian felt her toes just barely graze it. "I remember thinking, 'This is not happening! Why now?'" recalls Isaković. "Then, in a split second, I was able to refocus." Riding a surge of adrenaline, she tore down the last length to nab a silver medal, breaking the previous world record and missing gold by just 0.15 seconds.

Olympic athletes are strong and fit and tough. But none of that matters if they're not also resilient, capable of shaking off setbacks and adapting quickly to unexpected circumstances. When I met Isaković in 2013, she was a research assistant at the University of California, San Diego, working with a neuroscientist and psychiatrist named Martin Paulus to identify the neural characteristics that separate elite endurance performers from the rest of us—the mental skills that allowed her to regroup instead of crumble in Beijing. "We usually think along the lines of how you make someone less bad," Paulus explained to me. "Instead, we're asking whether we can use neuroscience, and brain imaging in particular, to understand how to make the brain work better."

Paulus came to UCSD from Germany in 1986, and he rapidly adjusted to the California lifestyle (though he recently accepted a cross-appointment at the Laureate Institute for Brain Research, in Oklahoma). He's an avid cyclist, with the notably calm demeanor of someone who has been practicing Zen meditation for three decades—"I get up at 5:00," he says, "and I hit the cushion by 5:10." A major strand of his research has focused on the role of interoception—the brain's monitoring of internal signals in the body like temperature, hunger, blood-oxygen levels, and so on—in anxiety disorders and addiction. Anxious people, he found, tend to overreact to negative stimuli, producing a distinct pattern of brain activity. Elite endurance, athletes, on the other hand, display a completely opposite response pattern. Was there a way, he wondered, of training the brains of the former to look more like the latter?

On a bright fall day, Isaković led me across the UCSD campus from Paulus's lab to a building where the group's research volunteers come for brain imaging. The protocol involves climbing into the cylindrical bore of a giant three-Tesla magnet for functional MRI scanning, which detects subtle changes in oxygen use to identify which areas of the brain are tackling different tasks. While they're in the claustrophobia-inducing confines of the fMRI, the subjects complete some simple cognitive tests similar to the ones Marcora uses, all the while breathing through a special tube. The twist: periodically and without warning, the flow of oxygen through the tube is restricted, temporarily making it difficult (but not impossible) to breathe. The volunteer on the day I visited was taking part in a study of teen drug users, which was looking for telltale patterns in their response to this stressful "aversive stimulus."

Paulus and his colleagues have found that crucial differences show up in the activation of the insular cortex, a region of the brain that monitors sensory signals from within the body. In a series of studies starting in 2012, the researchers put hardened marines, elite adventure racers, and ordinary people through the fMRI tests. Some members of the control groups panicked and had to be removed from the scanner, but the elite performers handled the scenario with ease. In fact, while the control groups got worse at the cognitive task when their breathing was restricted, the elite groups actually got *better*—precisely the sort of performance under stress that enables you to dig a little deeper when the stakes are highest, whether in the heat of combat or at the end of a multi-day adventure race.

Before the breathing restriction starts, the athletes already have higher levels of activity in their insular cortex—consistent with the idea that they've become adept at monitoring their own signals. "Typically, athletes are pretty in tune with their body awareness," Lori Haase, another of Paulus's colleagues, told me. They're in a state of watchful anticipation, ready to handle any discomfort that arises. Then, when the flow of air is restricted and the discomfort begins, the situation flips: insular cortex activity stays low in the athletes, but goes haywire in the controls and in people with anxiety and related problems.

Paulus draws a direct link between these findings and the research of Noakes and others on the importance of perceived effort in endurance. First, heightened internal awareness allows elite endurance athletes to anticipate and prepare for unpleasantness, avoiding the all-important mismatch between expected and actual effort described by Tucker. Then, subduing the natural reaction (or overreaction) to discomfort—what Marcora calls response inhibition—allows them to push on.

So how do you train your insular cortex? The approach that Paulus came up with reflects his Buddhist leanings. After all, the internal awareness that characterizes elite endurance athletes sounds a lot like the Buddhist concept of mindfulness, which in recent years has emerged as a mainstream fad with bestselling apps and wide-ranging claims about its curative powers for everything from depression to the common cold. The extraction of mindfulness from its Buddhist context began in the 1970s, when a University of Massachusetts researcher and Zen student named Jon Kabat-Zinn began developing what became a standardized eight-week "mindfulness-based stress reduction" course. The goal, Paulus explains, is to cultivate "nonjudgmental self-awareness": for a marathoner, leg pain and shortness of breath become neutral sources of information, to be used for pacing, rather than emotionally charged warnings to panic about. "You learn to monitor how your body actually feels, while suspending judgment about it," he says.

As with Marcora's brain training ideas, the first interest in Paulus's plans came from the military. His location, in San Diego, gives him easy access to collaborators at the Naval Health Research Center, as well as to marines training at nearby Camp Pendleton, and special forces troops, including Navy SEALs, across San Diego Bay at Naval Amphibious Base Coronado. In one study, published in 2016, a group led by Paulus and Haase's colleague Douglas Johnson, of UCSD and the Naval Health Research Center's Warfighter Performance Department, followed eight Marine infantry platoons during training prior to deployment to Afghanistan. Half the platoons received a specially modified version of Kabat-Zinn's eight-week mindfulness training, to see if the brain patterns of the raw recruits could be altered to make them more like the hardened Navy SEALs and elite endurance athletes the researchers had previously tested. Sure enough, while brain scans in the training-as-usual platoons showed the usual panicked leap in insular cortex activity when breathing restriction kicked in, the mindfulness-trained marines instead reduced their insular cortex activity. The hope, though this remains to be tested, is that this heightened resilience to stress will help the soldiers handle the inevitable chaos they will encounter during combat and reduce their likelihood of developing post-traumatic stress disorder.

The demands facing athletes are, of course, different from those encountered by soldiers, so Haase and Paulus, working with collaborators from the UCSD Center for Mindfulness, decided to develop a program tailored specifically for sports performance. The result was mPEAK—Mindful Performance Enhancement, Awareness & Knowledge—another eight-week program modeled on Kabat-Zinn's stress-reduction course. This version of mindfulness training puts more emphasis on sport-specific skills like concentration and embracing rather than avoiding pain, and addresses common athlete pitfalls like perfectionism by teaching self-compassion. It also incorporates what Haase calls "experiential exercises," like breathing through a straw or holding your hand in a bucket of ice water for as long as you can.

To test the protocol, Haase teamed up with seven athletes from the U.S. Olympic BMX racing team, whose athletes compete in a series of intense, rough-and-tumble bike races over challenging courses with no margin for error. Once again, brain scans showed a shift to more optimal responses to stressful challenges like breath restriction, and the teaching sessions offered the athletes a chance to reflect on what goes on in their mind in these moments of stress. The superficial thoughts are obvious—"It's typically like, 'I can't breathe,' 'I need more air,' 'if I don't get more air I'm going to pass out,'" Haase says—but there's also an underlying narrative that determines how you react to those sensations, which can be either positive or negative. Subjectively, psychological tests showed that the BMX riders displayed greater awareness of bodily sensations, and the national team head coach noted improvements in their race performance. "Their body language is calmer in the gate," the coach said. "They move their hands less on the bars, and they get out of the gate a little faster."

For now, it's hard to classify either Marcora's or Haase and Paulus's brain training approaches as anything more than intriguing anecdotes. They're both based on well-researched concepts, but the road from theory to practice is littered with the smoking remains of countless heavily hyped ideas that didn't pan out. So we'll have to wait. In the meantime, Marcora is working with an app developer to make his brain endurance training protocol portable and easy to use. And Haase and her colleagues have run more tests on a high school lacrosse team, and submitted a proposal to deploy mPEAK for perhaps the greatest endurance challenge of all: testing potential Mars astronauts for NASA. It's an alluring thought—that "the right stuff" isn't, after all, something you have to be born with. Perhaps, with sufficient hard work and mental effort, you can train it.

Or maybe there's a shortcut.

CHAPTER 12

Zapping the Brain

A sharp bang, like the crack of a rifle, echoed off the walls of the converted warehouse. After a brief, shocked silence, everyone rushed to their bikes, checking to see whose tire had blown. Personally, I was more worried about the guy slumped in a dentist's chair at the far end of the room, dripping sweat and dangling wires, who was getting zapped by a brain stimulator that looked like a Ping-Pong paddle with two heads. I stowed the notebook where I'd been scribbling notes and headed over to find out. If we had just blown out Tim Johnson's brain, I didn't want to write about it.

I was at Red Bull's global headquarters, located in a low-slung industrial neighborhood in Santa Monica, California, for a boundary-pushing training camp-slash-science experiment that the company dubbed "Project Endurance." Five world-class cyclists and triathletes had flown in—voluntarily, as far as I knew—to be prodded, zapped, and repeatedly pushed to their limits by a multinational swarm of several dozen researchers who would measure their every twitch and palpitation. The big question they were hunting: What role does the brain play in setting our physical limits? And can we change those limits—break through to another level—by trickling a small electric current through the brain's motor cortex?

To find out, the energy drink company enlisted Dylan Edwards and David Putrino, a pair of Australian-born neuroscientists at the Burke Rehabilitation Center and Weill Cornell Medical College in New York, to devise a five-day testing protocol—three days at Red Bull headquarters in Santa Monica, two at the StubHub velodrome twenty miles down the 405 in Carson—using electric and magnetic brain stimulation, peripheral nerve stimulation, EMG, EEG, and an array of other measurement tools to tease apart the effects of central (in the brain) and peripheral (in the muscles) fatigue as the athletes were pushed to the breaking point again and again.

"I think of my brain as a tool," Johnson, a six-time national cyclo-cross champion, had been explaining to me a few minutes before the bang. Racing, he said, was as much a battle against the limits imposed by his mind as it was a contest with his competitors. Fortunately, the loud explosion hadn't inflicted any damage on his tool. If anything, it was the other way around: Johnson's brain had somehow blown a circuit in one of the brain stimulation machines. Testing halted for a few hours while a replacement machine was rushed into place, and I seized the opportunity to quiz Holden MacRae, a sports medicine professor at Pepperdine University who also serves as Red Bull's chief physiologist, about the project's ultimate goals.

"It's about the nature of fatigue," explained MacRae, a trim, straight-backed South African expat. "Why do we slow down? Why do we make that *decision* to slow down." MacRae had worked with—guess who?—Tim Noakes during his Ph.D. work in Cape Town in the late 1980s, studying the effects of endurance training on lactate production, and was heavily influenced by Noakes's ideas about the brain's role in exercise. But for Red Bull's quest to push limits and give its athletes an edge, the mere existence of the central governor theory wasn't the point, and nor was the sometimes esoteric debate between Noakes and Marcora. "We know there's something in the brain that regulates performance," MacRae said matter-of-factly. "Now we want to see if we can manipulate it."

People have been shocking their brains for fun and profit since long before anyone understood what electricity was. Scribonius Largus, the court physician for the Roman emperor Claudius more than two thousand years ago, recommended the application of a live torpedo fish—an electric ray capable of delivering up to 200 volts at a time—to the forehead for relief of headaches, and other cultures around the world prescribed electric fish for everything from epilepsy to exorcism. By the end of the eighteenth century, the great debate between Luigi Galvani and Alessandro Volta had introduced the idea of "animal electricity" to the world. Galvani's nephew Giovanni Aldini soon began using "galvanism" to treat depression in Bologna (as well as applying electricity to the brains of freshly decapitated criminals to elicit bizarre facial expressions). In the two centuries since then, various forms of electrical brain stimulation for mental health and other conditions have drifted in and out of fashion with decidedly mixed results.

These days, talk of electricity and the brain still tends to provoke comments about either Frankenstein (a book that was reputedly inspired, in part, by Aldini's public demonstrations) or *One Flew Over the Cuckoo's Nest*. "My first thought was 'How is this different from the electroshock therapy they did in the 50s,'" admitted Rebecca Rusch, an ultra-distance mountain biker who was the first Red Bull athlete in the dentist's chair that morning. "I was like, they're going to do *what* to my head?" But the technique Edwards and Putrino had in mind, known as transcranial direct current stimulation, or tDCS, is very different, so Rusch had eventually come around to the idea, lured by the promise of learning more about the hidden reserves she relies on to win races. "If you're being chased by a lion, or a car falls on a baby, you find something extra," she said. "I think we're just touching the iceberg of 'How do we train that?'"

From a functional perspective, the brain is basically a giant electric circuit—a vast web of interconnected neurons that communicate with each other by firing electric discharges. The relatively strong currents applied in electroshock (or, as it's now known, electroconvulsive) therapy trigger all the affected neurons to fire at once, causing a seizure. In tDCS, the current is 500 to 1,000 times smaller—too small to directly cause the neurons to fire. Instead, sustaining this small trickle of current for ten to twenty minutes alters the sensitivity of the neurons, making them slightly more likely to fire (or, if you run the current in the opposite direction, slightly less likely to fire). The current, on its own, does nothing—but it primes your brain to respond differently to whatever happens next.

The technique is disarmingly—almost disturbingly—simple to administer: you connect a voltage source (a 9-volt battery will do) to two electrodes placed on opposite sides of your head. The precise placement of the electrodes determines which regions of your brain the current flows through. And there's no question that tDCS can have real effects. Between 2013 and 2016 alone, researchers published more than two thousand studies exploring the technique's potential for goals as varied as enhancing learning, fighting addiction and depression, and improving walking ability in patients with neurological diseases. One report describes significant improvement in "trunk peak velocity" during tango dancing in a seventy-nine-year-old Argentinian man with moderate Parkinson's; in another report, soldiers improved their ability to spot snipers in a virtual-reality simulation.

There's also no question, though, that tDCS hype has long since diverged from what researchers (or the vibrant DIY tDCS community) have actually demonstrated, triggering a skeptical backlash. At a conference in 2016, György Buzsáki, of New York University, presented results from a cadaver study showing that only about 10 percent of the electric current that is applied to a skull even makes it into the brain, prompting one tDCS researcher to describe the field as "a sea of bullshit and bad science." So, as I watched the proceedings at Red Bull, I filtered my impressions through a veil of skepticism. Yes, it seemed reasonable that electricity could alter brain function—but to enhance endurance, you would need to know exactly which part of the brain sets your limits.

A few weeks after the London Olympics in 2012, I was in Zurich to cover the Weltklasse track meet, the traditional season-ending supermeet that has hosted more than two dozen world records over the years.

But I skipped the morning media events with Usain Bolt and other stars, opting instead to hop onto a tram that took me to a satellite campus of the University of Zurich in a northern suburb of the city. I had arranged to meet a neuropsychologist named Kai Lutz, who was pioneering a new approach to the study of endurance. For years, researchers like Noakes had speculated about what might be happening in the brain at the moment of exhaustion. Lutz, who had spent fifteen years acquiring expertise in advanced neuroimaging, had a seemingly radical notion: why not take a look inside to find out?

To be fair, looking inside the brain during exercise is a daunting technical challenge, and even now it can only be done under very specific—and, critics would say, unnatural—conditions. The bike-in-an-MRI machine that Noakes showed me, which involved lying on your back in a magnet bore while pedaling a driveshaft, hasn't yet yielded any significant insights. Lutz, whose interest in the limits of endurance was initially spurred by his brain-imaging studies on the mysteries of tooth pain, took a more cautious and methodical approach. A soft-spoken and meticulous German researcher who had moved to Switzerland after completing his Ph.D., he started with a relatively simple experiment in which volunteers were tested on hand-grip strength. They repeated a series of thirteen-second contractions, with the required strength carefully manipulated so that they would fail to hold it about half the time. Functional MRI scans showed that two regions of the brain, the insular cortex and the thalamus, were more active during the failed contractions. The results made sense, since—as Martin Paulus's resilience studies, described in the previous chapter, also found—the insular cortex monitors incoming signals from the rest of the body. "It's not just muscle signals," Lutz notes. "The insular cortex is also involved in the emotional response of hearing your heart pound and so on."

MRI scans are great for pinpointing what regions of the brain are involved in a given activity, but they're less useful for figuring out what each region is actually doing. The main problem is that they're slow: to get decent resolution, you need two or three seconds per scan.

And they're also indirect measures of brain activity: they measure the changes in blood flow in different regions of the brain, which happen *after* you use that part of the brain. In contrast, you can use electroencephalography—better known as EEG—to listen directly to the electrical activity in the brain in real time, although the data is messier and harder to interpret. "The first study used MRI to figure out where to look," Lutz explained—and that enabled them to zero in for a more detailed investigation with EEG.

In the EEG study, volunteers strapped on what looked like a shower cap dotted with 128 silver electrodes to measure their brain activity, then rode a stationary bike for thirty to forty minutes until they reached exhaustion. They had to keep their heads as still as possible, staring straight ahead at a sheet of paper with a cross on it to avoid making eye movements that would throw the EEG measurements off. With the heightened time sensitivity of the EEG data, a telltale pattern emerged in the data. Shortly before the cyclists gave up, there was an increase in communication between the insular cortex, which was monitoring their internal condition, and the motor cortex, which issued the final commands to their leg muscles. The brain, in other words, knew that the cyclists were about to reach their limits *before* their legs actually failed, seemingly demonstrating Noakes's anticipatory regulation in action.

Lutz's doctoral student, who was running the study, sent an email to Noakes saying, in essence, "Look, we've found the central governor!"

For anyone interested in the athletic potential of brain stimulation, Lutz's results, which were published in late 2011, painted a bright target on two areas in the brain: the insular cortex and the motor cortex. Suppress the excitability of neurons in the insular cortex—the site of Lutz's central governor—and you might turn down the insular cortex's brake signal, allowing the motor cortex to keep driving the muscles for a little longer. Or, alternately, enhance motor cortex excitability and you might enable those neurons to simply ignore the brake signal and keep firing.

The latter approach, stimulating the motor cortex, had already been explored in a relatively obscure study published four years earlier by Alberto Priori, an Italian researcher at the University of Milan who was one of the pioneers of tDCS. He found that a ten-minute bout of tDCS to the motor cortex boosted endurance by about 15 percent in a sustained contraction of the elbow flexors (the muscles you use in a biceps curl) compared to when the volunteers received sham stimulation—support, seemingly, for the idea that brain stimulation can amplify the output from the motor cortex in the face of fatigue.

And it didn't take long, following the publication of Lutz's results, for researchers to try stimulating the insular cortex. In 2015, a Brazilian group led by Alexandre Okano of the Federal University of Rio Grande do Norte published the results of a brain stimulation test on ten national-class cyclists. This time, the cyclists received twenty minutes of tDCS to the temporal and insular cortices—an inevitable consequence of brain structure, since current has to flow through the temporal cortex to reach the insular cortex underneath it. In a progressively accelerating ride to exhaustion, the cyclists increased their peak power by about 4 percent when they received real tDCS compared to the sham stimulation used as a placebo. Strikingly, their rating of perceived effort was lower right from the beginning of the cycling test—a finding consistent with the idea that the insular cortex monitors signals from throughout the body and assesses their significance.

It's tempting to see these results as puzzle pieces that fit neatly into a coherent picture of how the brain controls endurance—after all, the fact that the insular cortex keeps turning up in these studies is awfully suggestive. But the full story is likely more complicated. For example, Okano's subjects also showed changes in heart rate, suggesting that stimulation had altered the function of the central nervous system. tDCS is, after all, a blunt tool: it's impossible to limit stimulation to a single brain area, since the current has to flow from one electrode to the other through multiple brain regions. When I asked Priori how he interpreted his own results, he too was reluctant to paint a simple picture of tDCS either suppressing input to the brain or enhancing output: it's likely a mix of both, he said.

So let's hold off, for now, on drawing any conclusions on exactly how a putative central governor might work. These initial results suggest some promising avenues for researchers to pursue as brain imaging and stimulation technology improves; further studies, meanwhile, have implicated other brain areas in the regulation of endurance, including the prefrontal cortex (which seems to get starved of oxygen as physical exhaustion approaches) and the anterior cingulate cortex (which is closely tied to the perception of effort). To Kai Lutz, whose EEG research pointed a finger at the insular cortex, all these possibilities are not mutually exclusive. Instead, he sees motivation, effort, and pain as distinct but interrelated factors that influence endurance through separate "processing loops" between various brain regions. The firmest conclusion from Priori's and Okano's studies, in the end, is something simpler but no less powerful: a proof of principle that, when it comes to manipulating the brain to enhance endurance, something, somehow, seems to work. And that, not surprisingly, was enough to get the attention of the sports world.

"There's at least 17 devices stuck to my body right now, if I'm counting correctly," said Jesse Thomas, an ultra-distance triathlete who had flown in from his home in Oregon for the Red Bull project. "And that doesn't even count the brain stuff—there's another 30 wires there." Thomas was surrounded by a swarm of scientists and technicians who were wiring him up for another series of maximal exercise tests, which would culminate with a four-kilometer all-out time trial on the stationary bike. In addition to the brain stimulation, Red Bull's scientific team was measuring a bewildering array of variables, from blood and urine samples to brain waves to leg angles to oxygen saturation in

his muscle cells. "If you take a step back and imagine yourself floating above and looking down on all this, it's actually pretty funny,"
Thomas acknowledged. "How did we get to this point?"

Red Bull's ethos of extreme adventure and boundary-pushing ap-
plies as much to its high-performance research program as it does to
its athletes and advertising (all of which are, of course, intertwined).
Felix Baumgartner's record-breaking skydive from the stratosphere,
in which he reached a supersonic speed of 833.9 miles per hour, was a
perfect illustration of how the company likes to mix stunt and science.
They've also made a habit of bringing together top athletes from various sports and pushing them in novel ways—sending surfers, skiers,
and snowboarders to Hawaii to learn freediving and breath-holding
skills, for example. Similarly, the brain-stimulation camp was as much
about convincing the athletes that they were capable of more than
they realized as it was about the science.

Still, Edwards and Putrino, the Australian neuroscientists, were
determined to seize the opportunity to collect some unique data—and
in doing so, to highlight the link between athletic training and physical rehabilitation from conditions like brain and spinal cord injuries,
which is their primary research interest. "Rehab and high-intensity
training are not as different as people believe," Putrino said. "Whether
you're a high-end athlete or a patient fighting locked-in syndrome,
you're dealing with the same limitations of muscle fatigue." Research
into the use of tDCS to help paralyzed patients in the long and arduous process of relearning to walk had been spurred, in part, by
Priori's 2007 study of motor cortex stimulation, so Edwards and Putrino elected to try a similar protocol on the athletes. "Our brains are
sending signals to our muscles; as we fatigue, those signals are getting weaker and weaker," Putrino explained. "The brain is making a
choice. But the brain's opinion isn't always right."

One of the key elements of the experiment was that the athletes
would only get real brain stimulation half the time. They would go
through all the motions before each of the six all-out four-kilometer
time trials that they completed over four days, first in the controlled

lab environment at Red Bull headquarters, and then at the velodrome. But half the time, the current would be turned off after a minute. To demonstrate, Edwards wired me up in a neoprene cap embedded with eight electrodes, then ramped up the current. I briefly felt the faint sensation of thousands of very small ants crawling on my scalp, but it quickly faded and I soon couldn't tell whether the current was on or off. (In fact, even after I'd taken the cap off, I kept imagining I still felt the ants.) So, for any given time trial, the athletes had no way of knowing whether their brains were juiced or not; only the stopwatch would, in theory, tell.

In March 2016, James Michael McAdoo, a power forward for the Golden State Warriors, tweeted out a photo of himself in the training room, sporting a pair of slick over-the-ear headphones. Though you couldn't tell from the picture, these particular headphones incorporated a miniature fakir's bed of soft plastic spikes above each ear, pressing gently into the skull and delivering pulses of electric current to the brain. Made by a Silicon Valley start-up called Halo Neuroscience, the headphones promised to "accelerate gains in strength, explosiveness, and dexterity" through a proprietary technique called neuropriming—a slightly modified version of tDCS. "Thanks to @HaloNeuro for letting me and my teammates try these out!" McAdoo tweeted. "Looking forward to seeing the results!"

As the basketball season wore on, the Warriors rolled over opponents with unprecedented ease, eventually finishing with a new regular-season record of 73 wins and just 9 losses. No one attributed their success to Halo's tDCS headphones (which, a trainer for the team confirmed, an unspecified number of players had experimented with)—but the high-tech device fit in with the team's techno-utopian storyline. Since the then-bumbling Warriors franchise was purchased by a group of Silicon Valley venture capitalists, in 2010, it has acquired a reputation as "tech's team," playing with the wonky, numbers-driven approach of Sand Hill Road venture capitalists. The Warriors have also been enthusiastic early adopters of technology ranging from "intelligent sleep masks" for countering jet lag to body-worn sensors that detect pressure on the knees and ankles. Now they were among the first to try brain stimulation—and, as their rivals (not to mention fans and amateur athletes) couldn't help noticing, they were winning a lot of games.

Halo was founded in 2013 by Daniel Chao and Bret Wingeier, who had previously worked together at a company that used another form of brain stimulation to treat epilepsy. Their headphones are designed to work in much the same way that Red Bull tried with cyclists (not coincidentally, Andy Walshe, Red Bull's director of high performance, is prominently listed as an advisor on Halo's website): the electrodes are positioned to trickle current through the motor cortex, and you can adjust the settings to focus on the brain regions associated with upper-body muscles, lower-body muscles, or both, depending on your intended activity. Don the headphones for twenty minutes during your warm-up, activate them with the associated app, and your brain will learn to deliver "stronger, more synchronous" signals to your muscles, the company claims.

While Priori's and Okano's studies generated a surge of interest in tDCS for sports, subsequent results have been mixed. In early 2017, a team at the University of Kent's Endurance Research Group, led by Alexis Mauger, reviewed the existing literature on how tDCS affects endurance (which they defined as continuous exercise lasting longer than 75 seconds). The ten other studies they located were all published in 2013 or later, and the protocols they used were all over the map: different stimulation times, currents, electrode placements, exercises, and so on. Overall, eight of twelve studies showed improved performance, while four saw no change. Halo has conducted its own unpublished pilot studies with groups like the U.S. ski team, claiming impressive improvements in propulsive force for ski jumpers after repeated use in training, for example—but without a properly blinded placebo control group. The company says it plans to submit research to peer-reviewed journals, but its initial strategy relied on a familiar

Silicon Valley script, distributing the device to high-profile athletes like McAdoo and hoping for good word of mouth.

It's difficult, then, to make any sort of informed judgment about Halo's headphones. When I wrote about them for the *New Yorker,* as Golden State attempted to clinch a second consecutive NBA title, I concluded that at worst they functioned as an industrial-strength placebo—a gadget with real (if disputed) science behind it, whose benefits are *supposed* to be all in your head. Golden State lost anyway, to LeBron James's Cleveland Cavaliers. But when Halo called and offered to lend me a pair for a month to try for myself, I decided—despite my long-standing distrust of subjective gear reviews—to give it a shot. By wiring myself up with a GPS watch, heart-rate monitor, and high-tech multi-axial accelerometer to analyze my stride parameters, I figured I might be able to detect whether brain stimulation had any measurable impact on my running.

I should pause here to explain that, as a journalist who covers sports science and technology, I am inundated on a near-daily basis with offers to try out new products, ranging from delicious-sounding energy bars to insanely complicated electro-adaptive T-shirt/running coach/ stride analyzers. I invariably decline, because my goal is to write about whether things work, not whether I like them—and for me, the former goal feels easier when I don't have an opinion about the latter. I want data, not feelings. So agreeing to trial the Halo headphones was a big departure for me—one that reflects the unusually strong interest aroused by the idea of brain stimulation. The prospect that you might be able to unlock your body's hidden reserves of endurance simply and painlessly by running a few electrons through a carefully selected part of your brain fascinated me. It felt like the culmination of a search that had spanned more than two decades, since that night in Sherbrooke when a linguistic misunderstanding had somehow unlocked my potential as a 1,500-meter runner.

Except that it wasn't painless. The headphones come with three electrode pads, each with 24 little foam spikes that you soak in saline solution before each use to make good electrical contact with your head. But I'm bald, and apparently the harsh Canadian climate has toughened my scalp to an unusual degree. In order to get the green light indicating that the electrodes had achieved contact, I had to press the headphones so hard that I would get deep divots across the top of my head. Sometimes I couldn't make contact at all, and when I did, turning on the current elicited a fierce burning sensation even on the lowest setting. On the rare occasions that I managed to endure twenty minutes of neuropriming, I was so frustrated and uncomfortable that, if anything, I felt worse when I finally headed out the door to run. This, I should emphasize, is precisely the sort of subjective experience that doesn't tell us much about whether the technique works. But I was glad I hadn't spent $750 on it.

What will it mean if brain stimulation really works? One obvious specter is brain doping, a possibility that Alexandre Okano acknowledged when I asked him about the implications of his research. The technique will lead to "benefits comparable to using drugs," he said. And "there is no known way to detect reliably whether or not a person has recently experienced brain stimulation." The safety risks of tDCS are thought to be minimal (though some researchers point out the lack of long-term studies, especially on the developing brains of young people), but the ethics of brain boosting will nonetheless require plenty of debate. Personally, my gut instinct is to hope that anti-doping authorities proactively ban the technique before it becomes widespread, simply because I'm uncomfortable with imagining my sixteen-year-old self, desperate for any athletic edge, playing around with scalp-mounted electrodes. But I fully understand that others might disagree with banning an apparently safe and noninvasive way of boosting performance.

To researchers like Alexis Mauger, tDCS is interesting as a research tool rather than a competitive aid. Just as, in his earlier studies, he used Tylenol to boost endurance in order to demonstrate the importance of pain, tDCS offers an unprecedented tool to probe the role of different sensations and brain regions in regulating endurance. And on a practical level, Mauger's most recent research hints at a potential methodological breakthrough as well as an explanation for the current mess of seemingly conflicting results. Most tDCS studies place both electrodes on the skull, which means you enhance the excitability of neurons under the negative electrode but suppress the excitability of those under the positive electrode. So the benefits that one electrode giveth, the other may taketh away, depending on exactly where it's placed. As an alternative, Mauger tried placing the positive electrode on the shoulder instead of the skull while stimulating the motor cortex. The results were immediately encouraging: a reduction in perceived effort accompanied by a 23 percent increase in time to exhaustion on the bike with the shoulder electrode, compared to no change in either parameter when both electrodes were on the skull.

Still, translating lab research into a real-world competitive context remains a formidable barrier. This challenge was on my mind on my fourth day in California, when the Red Bull cyclists, trailed by their entourage of scientists, headed to the StubHub velodrome for a final round of testing. Away from the controlled environment of the lab and its futile stationary bikes, it was easier to connect the dry clinical discussions of "maximal voluntary contraction" and "task failure" with the messy reality of no-holds-barred competition. On the first four-kilometer time trial of the day, Tim Johnson, the cyclocross champion, notched the fastest time with a 5:20. Jesse Thomas, the ultra-distance triathlete, was just two seconds back. A few hours later, after another round of brain stimulation, Thomas managed to drop his time to 5:10, then stood on the sidelines cheering as Johnson, wheels tracing a perfectly level contour around the steep curves, tried to reclaim the throne.

Stopwatches clicked as Johnson whizzed past the finish in 5:17. "Did I get him?" he panted as he circled past the finish line again a moment later. Thomas laughed, savoring the triumph. "That's the first thing I asked when I finished too. It's the same mindset." He glanced around at the hundreds of thousands of dollars' worth of machinery arrayed on the infield, the laptops and transmitters, the sensors and wires poking out of his bike shorts. "You can do all this shit, but it all comes down to two guys on a bike, trying to beat each other."

I've thought a lot about brain stimulation since then—its potential as a research tool, its hasty and (as far as my scalp is concerned, at least) premature commercialization, its likely impact on the acceptable boundaries of athletic self-improvement—and Thomas's comments have stuck with me. Because the morning after his battle with Johnson, before heading to the airport, I cornered one of the scientists and asked for a peek at the randomization protocol. In each of the two races, it turned out, the winner had received sham stimulation while the loser had received the real thing. You can't draw any conclusions about whether tDCS "works" from a single anecdote, but it nonetheless felt like a hype-dousing splash of cold water.

Maybe, I reflected, the electrodes are beside the point. From Red Bull's perspective, the goal of bringing its athletes together for these camps, whether for brain stimulation or breath-hold training, is to teach athletes that they're capable of more than they think. Brain stimulation may or may not turn out to be an effective way of *accessing* your hidden reserves, but there was little doubt that the athletes at the camp came away from the experience convinced that these reserves exist. In the end, when it comes down to two guys on a bike, maybe that's the real secret weapon: *believing* that you have another gear.

CHAPTER 13

Belief

I spent the evening before the 2003 Cherry Blossom 10-Mile Run poring obsessively over the list of elite entrants. There were about two dozen names on the men's list, the vast majority of them from Kenya, vying for a share of the $30,000 prize pot offered by the venerable Washington, D.C., mega-race. Though I had plenty of experience with track and cross-country races, this was my first serious foray into the big-money world of road racing. The top twelve finishers would get cash—and, as I scrolled through the names and googled their past accomplishments, I suspected I would be right on the bubble.

The next morning, I set off from the blossom-strewn National Mall with fifteen thousand other runners. The elite group quickly separated themselves from the throng behind them, but the real racing didn't start right away. For the first two miles, everyone waited and watched, clipping their strides and listening to the rasp of their competitors' breathing. Finally, the Kenyan pair of John Korir and Reuben Cheruiyot, who between them had won the last three editions of the race, hit the front. The pace surged; the nervous energy of the tightly bunched pack was exhaled, and the race was on.

In a sense, every stride you take during a race is a microdecision: will you speed up, slow down, or maintain your current pace? But some decisions are more consequential than others. As Korir and Cheruiyot telescoped away, leaving the shrapnel of the exploded lead pack in their wake, I had to decide how hard to chase. I wasn't concerned about pace or splits; I had logged enough miles on the razor's edge, over the previous decade, to be able to feel in my gut precisely what was sustainable and what wasn't. I was as fit as I had ever been, and—let's be honest—wanted cash; but I was also disciplined and pragmatic. As the runners around me abruptly launched into what seemed like a near-sprint, I accelerated more steadily, hoping to hit the maximum pace I could sustain for the eight remaining miles. Soon all two dozen runners in the lead pack were receding into the distance in front of me. But I hoped to see at least some of them again.

My memories of the second half of that race are still vivid—the thrill of the hunt as, one by one, I began to track down and pass the stragglers. Some of them put up a brave fight. Others were barely jogging; you could almost see the metaphorical cloud of black smoke billowing from their overheated engines. Late in the race, I caught Simon Rono, a Kenyan who a few years earlier had notched the second-fastest winning time in the race's history, to move into twelfth place. I was in the money! With a few hundred yards remaining, some friends cheering on the sidelines pointed up the road to another Kenyan runner wobbling toward the finish. I lowered my head and charged, edging him just before the line to increase my payout from $200 to $250.

For years afterward, I told that story as a tale of triumph—a humble-brag about my finely honed pacing acumen. Knowing my limits and racing within them had allowed me to beat half the elite runners in the race. The others, I assumed, were simply faster than me, and I wouldn't have beaten them under any circumstances. It wasn't until almost a decade later, after many similar racing experiences, that I finally began to question that narrative.

Reid Coolsaet was wide awake, sprawled the wrong way on his hotel bed so that he could prop his legs up against the headboard. It was the night before the 2011 Toronto Waterfront Marathon, and outside the window a strong breeze scudded briskly along the exposed lakefront boulevard where, the next morning, he would try to run a qualifying time for the London Olympics. The gears of his mind spun restlessly, cranking out the mental arithmetic of kilometer splits for different paces and different scenarios: 2:11:29 to qualify; 2:10:09, or 3:05 per kilometer, to erase Jerome Drayton's thirty-six-year-old Canadian record. In training, he had drummed that pace into his mind and legs until it felt automatic.

As at Cherry Blossom, the front of the pack would be dominated by East African runners, mostly Kenyan and Ethiopian, aiming for a time several minutes faster than Drayton's record. They were irrelevant to Coolsaet. His only adversary, whether for fulfilling his Olympic dreams or collecting a $36,000 bonus for breaking the record, was the clock.

But something didn't feel quite right. Finally, he pulled out his earbuds, climbed out of bed, and padded downstairs to the hotel bar, where his longtime coach, Dave Scott-Thomas, was having a beer. "I want to go out with the leaders tomorrow," he said. "And I want you to tell me if that's insane or not." Scott-Thomas had been working with Coolsaet since 1998, shepherding him in gradual increments from mediocre university walk-on to world-class distance runner. Methodical planning and realistic goal-setting formed the bedrock of their coach-athlete relationship. But beneath Coolsaet's apparent uncertainty, Scott-Thomas sensed a seam of hard-earned confidence. "Why not?" he said, nodding. "Go for it!" With months of strategizing abruptly discarded, Coolsaet headed upstairs, crawled back into bed, and fell peacefully asleep within minutes.

The next morning, the race started with the usual exuberance, thousands of runners surging across the start line and down University Avenue like lava from a long-plugged volcano. I was leaning out the window of a press truck driving 40 or 50 meters ahead of the field, watching as the front-runners began to coalesce into distinct packs: the East Africans in the lead, then the Canadian Olympic hopefuls, followed by the top women, the top regional runners, and so on. As the miles ticked past, I started to exchange puzzled glances and raised eyebrows with a few other reporters. An eleven-man lead pack formed a ragged arrowhead across the road. Ten of the men were from Kenya and Ethiopia, but clearly visible at the back of the pack was an incongruous shock of red hair. As the runners streaked past a banner indicating the 5K mark, Coolsaet glanced down at his watch, clicked a button, and carried on running with the leaders. The torrid start wasn't a mistake, we realized: Coolsaet had abandoned the careful pacing plan he had outlined at the pre-race press conference a few days earlier, and was running to win.

By this time, I was fully accustomed to the typical patterns of road racing: the kamikaze attacks of the East Africans at the front of the pack, and the sober caution of the North American chasers. I assumed that the differences—a broad but not universal generalization, admittedly—could be attributed to simple economics. I once spent time with a manual-laborer-turned-runner named Joseph Nderitu, who told me about his first year racing in North America, when he managed to return home with $600 in his pocket, enough to buy two calves. The following year, after an even better season, he bought a quarter acre of land for $2,500, built a five-room house, and bought another cow—"the first cow for milking ever in my family," he told me with pride. For someone like me, running a personal-best time and placing sixth in a race where prize money was offered to the top five might be chalked up as a victory of sorts; for Nderitu, the self-actualization of a personal best would be a poor substitute for cash.

But to those who have actually spent time in Kenya and gotten to know the legions of aspiring runners there, this pat explanation doesn't capture the whole truth. Coolsaet, for example, regularly spent several months a year in Kenya, training with locals in the thin highland air. Even in training sessions, with nothing but pride on the line, he noticed that Kenyan and Western runners had markedly different mentalities. The Kenyan up-and-comers would simply run with the leaders—often international champions—for as long as possible, then drop out or start jogging when they could no longer keep up. Coolsaet and other foreigners, meanwhile, would maintain a steady but sustainable pace. At one point, he took some friends to watch the famous weekly fartlek workout in the hills around the town of Iten. More than two hundred runners streamed past them, raising a cloud of red dust from the dirt roads; about a third of them had dropped out of the workout before the halfway mark.

After hearing enough of these stories, I finally started to consider the obvious question. Given how good the Kenyans are, should I be emulating their racing style rather than laughing at it? There is, after all, something inherently limiting about the fetishization of "even pacing." If you execute a perfectly paced race, that means you effectively decided within the first few strides how fast you would complete the full distance. There is no opportunity to surprise yourself with an unexpectedly good day: you've put a ceiling on your potential achievement from the moment the starting gun fires. As a result, this approach may produce better results *on average*, but it is less likely to produce dramatic outliers: jaw-droppingly fast (or slow) times.

Looking back at my Cherry Blossom results, I see that I beat some blue-chip runners, like Simon Rono, the former champion, who would never have lost to me if they had raced more conservatively. But I also lost to some considerably less credentialed runners—another Kenyan named Francis Komu, for example—whose typical performances were pretty similar to my own. The difference in Komu's racing history is that, by racing aggressively, he now and then hit one out of the park, like he did that day in Washington when he beat me by a minute and a half. Instead of a consistent string of pretty good performance, he opted for a few great ones mixed in with some undeniable stinkers— which, when I thought about it, was a pretty good trade. And that, it seemed, was the choice Coolsaet was making in the Toronto marathon on that windy morning in 2011: when the leaders passed halfway on pace to run under 2:08, more than two minutes faster than the Canadian record and nearly three and a half minutes faster than Coolsaet's previous best, he was still tucked right behind them.

So if it's not just about money, why do Kenyans run the way they do? According to filmmaker and former elite runner Michael Del Monte, who spent months in the heart of Kenyan running culture while filming the documentary *Transcend* about the rise of marathoner-turned-politician Wesley Korir, it comes down to belief. Even the humblest

Kenyan runner, he noticed, wakes up every morning with the firm conviction that today, finally, will be his or her day. They run with the leaders because they think they can beat them, and if harsh reality proves that they can't, they regroup and try again the next day. And that belief, fostered by the longstanding international dominance of generations of Kenyan runners, becomes a self-fulfilling prophecy.

To sports scientists in an academic setting, *placebo* is a dirty word. The placebo effect is what skews the results of their experiments, and it's what allows charlatans to get rich peddling ineffective performance-boosters. But for those working with elite athletes in real-life settings, the picture is different. In 2013, physiologists Shona Halson and David Martin of the Australian Institute of Sport wrote an editorial in the *International Journal of Sports Physiology and Performance* in which they argued for a distinction between placebos and "belief effects"—valuable opportunities to improve athlete performance, which should be enhanced and harnessed rather than suppressed. After all, if a metaphorical sugar pill makes you faster and enables you to win a race, who cares if the effects were all in your head?

In fact, Halson and Martin argued, the boundary between "real" ergogenic (performance-enhancing) aids and "fake" belief effects is much fuzzier than most people, even scientists, realize. They cited an observation by sports scientist Trent Stellingwerff, who also coaches athletes including his wife, Hilary, a two-time Olympic 1,500-meter runner. At a conference in 2013, Stellingwerff noted the wide variety of supplements and training methods that have been shown to produce a 1–3 percent boost in performance, from caffeine to beet juice to altitude training. In theory, combining all these approaches should create a superathlete; in practice, studies that combine multiple interventions in elite athletes tend to see overall improvements of . . . 1 to 3 percent. If $1 + 1 + 1 = 1$, the implication is that many different "proven" training aids act, at least in part, on the same target: the brain.

That's not an argument in favor of sugar pills, Stellingwerff emphasizes. "For me, a placebo is direct trickery, giving an athlete an inert substance and saying it is something else. I've never done that, except in studies." Harnessing a belief effect, on the other hand, doesn't involve any trickery; rather, it's "very strategically and slowly developing maximal trust, belief, and evidence with your athletes and coaches over time." In the ideal scenario, he says, you're offering advice with real, evidence-backed physiological benefits, while bearing in mind that "the words you choose, how much info you provide, and how you describe it can all dictate the eventual performance impact of that intervention."

Consider the purported benefits of a post-workout ice bath, which is supposed to ward off inflammation and hasten muscle recovery. Athletes at every level swear by them; researchers, meanwhile, have published hundreds of studies investigating their effects, with results that are ambiguous at best. If you ask athletes how sore they feel the day after a workout, ice baths seem to help; if you take blood tests to look for objective signs of reduced muscle damage, not so much.

It's hard, of course, to have a "placebo-controlled" ice bath study, since you can't disguise the fact that you're immersing yourself in freezing water. But researchers at Australia's Victoria University found a way around this problem in a 2014 study. They compared fifteen-minute post-cycling-workout soaks in either cold water, lukewarm water, or lukewarm water with the addition of a special "recovery oil." "We made sure that we put the recovery oil in the water in plain sight of the participants," recalls David Bishop, the study's senior author, "and we gave them a glossy summary of some made-up research about scientifically proven benefits of 'recovery oils.'"

Over the following two days, the researchers tested their subjects' leg strength—which, in the end, is the most important recovery outcome. Sure enough, the ice bath significantly outperformed the lukewarm bath throughout the two-day recovery period. But the recovery oil was just as good, and perhaps even marginally better than the ice bath—even though the oil was, in fact, a liquid soap called Cetaphil Gentle Skin Cleanser. This, you might think, debunks the value of ice baths once and for all—except for the fact that the athletes who had either ice or oil really did seem stronger in the two days following the workout. Like Stellingwerff, Bishop sees the belief effect as a vital tool for coaches and sports scientists to harness. Liquid soap isn't a sustainable deception (eventually the athletes will start noticing how uncharacteristically good their teammates smell); ice baths, which have a plausible physiological role in fighting inflammation, can be recommended with a clean conscience.

If all this sounds like the sort of self-deluding rationalization you might expect to hear from some potion-peddling alternative medicine guru, rest assured I share your discomfort. I've written dozens of articles about ice bath research and still struggle with the appropriate message. My general take, these days, is that if you like ice baths and feel that they help you, you should stick with them. If you don't like them or haven't experienced them, there's no compelling reason you should start. I tend to be harsher on cryosaunas, the mini-chambers that dust you with a cloud of supercooled nitrogen vapor for a few minutes. The ambiguities in the research are similar, but spending tens of thousands of dollars on a placebo seems less defensible, though I recognize the inherent contradictions in my position.

It's also worth pointing out another flaw in the dichotomy between "real" and "fake" effects, which is that placebos can produce measurable biochemical changes. The paradigm-altering demonstration of this phenomenon came in a 1978 study, from the University of California, San Francisco, of people recovering from dental surgery. The patients were given IV drips of either morphine or a plain saline solution to block their pain; as expected, some "placebo responders" had reductions in pain even though they only received saline. The researchers then added a drug called naloxone, which counteracts overdoses of morphine and heroin by blocking the body's opioid receptors. This immediately shut off the painkilling effect of the saline solution, suggesting that its painkilling powers were the result of a surge of endorphins, the body's internal version of morphine.

And it's not just endorphins: subsequent research has shown many distinct signaling pathways that respond to placebo-driven expectations, including endocannabinoids, which are the body's internal version of cannabis, and the immune system. Coordinating all of these responses is the brain's anticipation and reward system, which depends on the neurotransmitter dopamine. As it happens, there's a gene called COMT that affects how much dopamine is available in the prefrontal cortex of your brain: those with one version of the gene have three to four times as much dopamine as those with the opposite version. Researchers at Harvard Medical School's Program in Placebo Studies, using sham acupuncture to treat irritable bowel syndrome, found that those with the high-dopamine version of the gene were far more likely to respond strongly to the placebo treatment—further evidence that those who do respond to placebos aren't merely imagining the effects.

What does all this have to do with the limits of endurance? On the simplest level, taking the equivalent of a sugar pill, if you really believe it will help you race faster, will often work. Chris Beedie, a researcher at Canterbury Christ Church University in Britain who studies placebos in sport, once had a group of cyclists complete a series of ten-kilometer time trials. The subjects were told they would receive various doses of caffeine before each trial, but they wouldn't be told which dose they had received. As expected, the cyclists rode 1.3 percent faster when they thought they had received a moderate dose, 3.1 percent faster after a high dose, and 1.4 percent *slower* when they thought they got the placebo. In reality, all the pills were placebos. The performance boost, and associated changes in how much pain or effort they perceived during the rides, were entirely fueled by their own expectations.

Similar belief effects can also show up with no pills in sight. For example, surveys have found that the greater your interest in sports, the more superstitious you're likely to be. Intrigued by all the tales of superstitious superathletes like Michael Jordan, who famously wore his old college shorts under his uniform throughout his professional career, German researcher Lynn Damisch of the University of Cologne set out to test whether lucky charms actually work. Sure enough, in one study, she found that simply saying "Here is your ball. So far it has turned out to be a lucky ball." boosted golf putting performance by 33 percent compared to saying "This is the ball that everyone has used so far." In other tasks, subjects set higher initial goals and tried for longer before giving up when they had their lucky charms with them—evidence that what psychologists call "self-efficacy," or a belief in their own competence and success, altered their behavior in ways that became self-fulfilling, like the aggressive racing of Kenyan runners.

So, yes, self-confidence can make you try harder—but it can also work in more subtle ways. Telling runners they look relaxed makes them burn measurably less energy to sustain the same pace. Giving rugby players a postgame debriefing that focuses on what they did right rather than what they did wrong has effects that continue to linger a full week later, when the positive-feedback group will have higher testosterone levels and perform better in the next game. Even doing a good deed—or simply imagining yourself doing a good deed—can enhance your endurance by reinforcing your sense of agency: in one study, donating a dollar to charity enabled volunteers to hold up a five-pound weight for 20 percent longer than they otherwise could. Worryingly, they gained even more strength from imagining themselves doing an evil deed—confirmation, perhaps, of a theory, long discussed on online running message boards, that the best way to run an 800-meter race is fueled by "pure hate."

This is not a suggestion that you should rob a convenience store on the way to your next race. Most of these examples, considered on their own, are little more than parlor tricks. Nevertheless, when you step back, a larger pattern comes into focus. When I was visiting Tim Noakes in Cape Town, I asked him what his theories about the brain's role in endurance could tell us about training. If there's a central governor, can you hone it? He answered me with an anecdote. During his days as a rower for the South African Universities team in the early

1970s, the crew regularly did a workout of six times 500 meters as hard as possible. "And one afternoon, we did our sixth and turned around to row back to the boathouse, and the coach says, 'No, go to the start again. You're doing another one.' So we did another 500. And he said go back. And we did another four. And you know, no one would have believed that we could do that, if you'd asked us." That lesson, he recalled, stuck with him—first as an athlete and later as a scientist: "You have to teach athletes, somewhere in their careers, that they can do more than they think they can."

This epiphany has a lot in common with what Amby Burfoot, a former Boston Marathon champion and longtime *Runner's World* editor, once described as the "absolute, no-doubt-in-the-world best running workout you can do." Burfoot was writing about a Yale University study in which the appetite hormones of a group of volunteers plunged after drinking what they were told was an "indulgent" high-calorie milk shake but didn't budge when they drank a "sensible" low-calorie shake—even though the two drinks were actually identical. The brain rules the body, Burfoot concluded, which is why his super-workout consisted of five times a mile as hard as possible, followed by your coach telling you to do another at the same pace. "From this workout, you'll learn forever that you're capable of much more than you think," he wrote. "It's the most powerful lesson you can possibly learn in running."

A vast body of sports-specific studies back this insight up, using various forms of deception to trick people into pushing harder or for longer than they normally can. Rigging the thermometer to display a falsely low temperature counteracts some of the endurance-sapping effects of heat. Using a clock that runs fast or slow, or lying about how much distance an athlete has covered, can help or hurt performance depending on the context. Several studies have used virtual reality systems to allow competitors to race against their own previous performances— a benchmark that, by definition, the subjects are confident they can match. This turns out to be true, even when the virtual rivals are secretly sped up, though only up to a point. Race against a 2-percent-improved version of yourself and you'll surprise yourself, a 2017 study from French researchers found; race against a 5-percent-improved version and you'll soon get discouraged when you realize you can't keep up.

But deception can take you only so far. Even if you have a coach who likes to play tricks on you, there's only so many times you'll fall for the old "extra interval" gag before you start holding back a bit in every workout. To Burfoot, the real point is more general. Deception, he writes, "is not central to the phenomenon—it just makes for compelling stories with surprise endings. What's central is strong belief."

Shortly after the halfway mark, Coolsaet began to drift behind the leaders. As he disappeared from our sight lines on the press truck, we shook our heads knowingly: confidence is great, but the marathon punishes overconfidence with Old Testament severity. So it was a surprise, a few miles later, to see him reappear in the distance. Head down, teeth gritted, he doggedly clawed his way back to the lead pack, which by the 30-kilometer mark was down to just six runners. In a live roadside interview on the TV race broadcast, his coach bluntly explained the temporary lapse: "He had to stop at about 22K to take a dump."

For Coolsaet, the strong belief that he could race with the Kenyans was earned by training with them. A few months after the Toronto race, back in the training mecca of Iten, high in the hills of the Rift Valley, he once again joined more than two hundred Kenyan runners, ranging from complete unknowns to established stars, for the weekly fartlek along the dusty mountain roads outside town. The task was simple: alternate two minutes hard with one minute easy and repeat twenty times. Just as in races, everyone went out hard and hung on for as long as they could. No one wanted to be behind the lone *mzungu*, but Coolsaet still managed to work his way up and finish near the front. As he jogged back toward town, caked in red dust and sweat, a handful of other runners burst into applause. He was ready to run

2:05, they told him—a vote of confidence with the energizing power of a wheelbarrow full of caffeine pills.

This sort of earned, transferable belief—if he can do it, so can I— also plays out at the very highest levels of sport. Why is it that world records in virtually every test of human endurance keep edging downward? You might think it's our ever-advancing knowledge of training, nutrition, hydration, recovery and so on, along with fancy technologies like cryosaunas. But all of this knowledge and technology is applied with equal enthusiasm to nonhuman sports like horse and dog racing. The financial stakes in horse racing, thanks to legalized betting, dwarf those in human endurance racing. And sure enough, for the first half of the twentieth century, Thoroughbreds and humans got faster at roughly similar rates. But according to a 2006 analysis by University of Nottingham researcher David Gardner, winning times at major races like the Kentucky Derby and the Epsom Derby have remained stagnant since about 1950. Over the same period, winning times at major marathons such as the Olympics continued to drop by more than 15 percent.

A champion marathoner and a champion horse are both physiological marvels; the difference is that the marathoner can look beyond the present moment. Secretariat's Kentucky Derby record of 1:59.4 has stood since 1973. Nearly thirty years later, in 2001, Monarchos became only the second horse to dip under 2:00 at the Derby, winning by five lengths. Could he have challenged Secretariat's record? Perhaps if Secretariat had been there in front of him. But only humans can make the abstract leap to virtual competition: if you know that someone, somewhere, has covered a given distance in 1:59.4, you know that it's *possible* to cover that distance in 1:59.3—and you can guide your training and execute your race plan accordingly.

Of course, believing you can run a 2:05 marathon isn't the same as running it. Philosophers make a distinction between justified beliefs and true beliefs. You can have a good reason for believing something (that your car is in the garage, for example) even if it turns out not to be true (because someone has stolen it). Conversely, you can be-lieve something that turns out to be true (that you will draw an ace) for no good reason. Knowledge, according to some philosophical ac-counts, requires justified true belief. For athletes, the simplest way of acquiring justified true belief about your capabilities is to test them: whatever you've done before, you can do again plus a little more. But the question raised by Noakes and Marcora and others is whether, for most of us, such incrementally justified beliefs understate our true capacities. To advance into uncharted territory—to, say, improve the marathon record by three minutes rather than three seconds, as Eliud Kipchoge hopes to do—requires an imaginative leap.

Just before the 35-kilometer mark, as the runners head up a short hill, Coolsaet surges into the lead. There are just four runners left in contention at this point. As Coolsaet presses ahead, 2:08 marathoner Nixon Machichim begins to drift back, losing contact with the group; later he drops out. For the remainder of the race, the runners have to push through a gusting headwind. Coolsaet's quads are burning and his stride starts to look slow and jerky. Finally, with just over two miles left to finish, his two remaining rivals—a 2:07 runner and a 2:05 runner—begin to pull away. As he falters in the wind, it becomes clear that he will miss the national record; but the journalists aboard the press truck are buzzing nonetheless. Despite the terrible conditions, he ends up running 2:10:55, for third place, to become the second-fastest Canadian in history and lock up a spot on the Olympic team—but it's how he did it, rather than the time itself, that sticks in my mind.

This book isn't a training manual. Still, it's impossible to explore the nature of human limits without wondering about the best ways to transcend them. In the end, the most effective limit-changers are still the simplest—so simple that we've barely mentioned them. If you want to run faster, it's hard to improve on the training haiku penned by Mayo Clinic physiologist Michael Joyner, the man whose 1991 journal paper foretold the two-hour-marathon chase:

Run a lot of miles
Some faster than your race pace
Rest once in a while

Joyner is one of the world's leading experts in the physiology of human endurance, but he gleefully describes himself as a "tech nudie." At one conference on the future of sports technology and performance enhancement, Joyner brought, as a prop, his vintage 1972 boxer's jump rope. All the blandishments of modern sports science—altitude tents and heart-rate-variability tracking and bioengineered sports drinks and so on—amount to minor tinkering compared to the more elemental task of pushing your mind and body in training, day after day, for years.

In fact, the very objectivity promised by sports technology turns out to be self-limiting in some contexts. Aiming to ride your bike at a specific target heart rate or power output is like even pacing on steroids: it reduces the risk of a blowup, but takes away the possibility of a breakthrough. As elite track coach Steve Magness has written, technological enhancements like running with a GPS watch "slacken the bond between perception and action." Ecological psychologists often use motorcycle riding as an illustration. You can monitor your speed by feeling the sensation of the bike and the rhythm of the road as the world flows past, or you can look at the speedometer. The latter is more precise, but for experts, at least, it's not a better way of assessing whether you're moving safely. Similarly, by checking your power meter before deciding whether to speed up or slow down when cycling, you're inserting an extra cognitive step that relies on an imperfect external estimate of how you should be feeling, rather than on the feeling itself.

So, if the basics of training are simple and widely understood, does all this research about the brain's hidden reserves teach us anything new? "I think all the great coaches always work on the brain anyway," Tim Noakes told me. But not everyone has a great coach, or any coach at all, for that matter. I really do think most of us can do a better job of accessing those "hidden reserves"; in particular, this is a relatively untapped area of improvement for those who are already training at a high level and possibly maxing out their potential for physical gains. Maybe approaches like brain training and brain stimulation will pan out, and deliver predictable and repeatable performance improvements. Or perhaps we'll have to rely on lower-tech ways of directly wrestling with our beliefs, like self-talk.

Of course, the power of belief has often been oversold, like the self-help books that claim sub-four-minute miles became easy as soon as Roger Bannister showed it was possible. In any honest accounting, training is the cake and belief is the icing—but sometimes that thin smear of frosting makes all the difference. Since Samuele Marcora's 2014 study showing that simple training in motivational self-talk could extend time to exhaustion in a cycling test, several other studies have confirmed that the technique can alter the relationship between pace and effort. A British field experiment found that self-talk training boosted performance in a grueling sixty-mile overnight ultramarathon. Stephen Cheung's research, described in Chapter 8, found that cyclists performed better in 95-degree heat after self-talk training that focused specifically on handling hot weather. If I could go back in time to alter the course of my own running career, after a decade of writing about the latest research in endurance training, the single biggest piece of advice I would give to my doubt-filled younger self would be to pursue motivational self-talk training—with diligence and no snickering.

In the end, though, what has captivated me about the new wave of brain-centered endurance research isn't really its performance-boosting potential. For millions of people around the world, endurance challenges are somewhere between a hobby and an addiction, a form of grueling self-test that has no particular health justification. Why? If races were really just plumbing contests—tests of whose pipes could deliver the most oxygen and pump the most blood—they would be boringly deterministic. You race once, and you know your limits. But that's not how it works.

As a college freshman on the track team, I once had a disheartening conversation with a girl on the basketball team whom I hoped to impress. She had an upcoming game, I had an upcoming meet, and we were discussing how nervous we were. "Why are you nervous?" she asked. "It's not like trying to hit a free throw in front of a screaming crowd. Isn't it just the gun goes, everybody runs, and whoever is fastest wins?" I tried to explain to her that every good race involved exceeding what felt like my physical limits. If I ran 800 meters as hard as I could in practice, I might run 2:10; in a race, I might run 1:55. Accessing that hidden reserve was anything but a foregone conclusion, and waiting to see how deep I would manage to dig was what made racing both exhilarating and terrifying. (I never did get a date with her.)

These days, the terror has mostly, though not entirely, faded. When I line up for a race, I remind myself that my fiercest opponent will be my own brain's well-meaning protective circuitry. It's a lesson I first learned in my breakthrough 1,500-meter race in Sherbrooke more than two decades ago, but its implications continue to surprise me. I'm eager to learn more, in the coming years, about which signals the brain responds to, how those signals are processed, and—yes— whether they can be altered. But it's enough, for now, to know that when the moment of truth comes, science has confirmed what athletes have always believed: that there's more in there—if you're willing to believe it.

Two Hours

May 6, 2017

T he thing about a two-hour marathon, under the heavily scripted
conditions that Nike has orchestrated, is that it should be almost
comically boring. If all goes well, there will be no surges, no breaks,
no comebacks, and not even the slightest variation in pace: just three
men, an arrowhead, and a clock. Despite these facts, the Breaking2
race appears to be the hottest unofficial ticket in Italy, even though it's
not open to the public. Samuele Marcora, who grew up in the town of
Busto Arsizio, twenty-five miles from Monza, is home looking after
his mother while on sabbatical from the University of Kent. I pull every string at my disposal to get him accredited as a media commentator, since I'm eager to hear his take in real time on this ultimate test of
endurance. It's not until 4 A.M. on the day of the race, which is slated
to start at 5:45 A.M., that I'm finally able to send him a message confirming that he's in. He replies immediately: "I was awake waiting for
your message. Couldn't sleep!!!"

In the predawn gloom, the bustle of final preparations at the Formula One track feels hushed and surreal. After a lengthy and sleepless
red-eye flight, a full day of deadline reporting, and a scant few hours
of rest, I've passed through the stage of feeling tired and instead am
pleasantly buzzed on adrenaline and Nutella-smeared croissants. I've
been telling people on Twitter who ask for predictions that I give Kipchoge and company a 1–10 percent chance of success; either that, or I
reply with a GIF of Clubber Lang from *Rocky III* saying "Prediction?
PAIN!" I have an all-too-familiar feeling in the pit of my stomach,

along with a leaden heaviness in my legs, that I know from long experience is not physical but mental. I'm having sympathy pains for Kipchoge, who is about to leap voluntarily into a chasm of unknown depths.

Once the race starts, it very quickly settles into a measured, seemingly effortless rhythm. After the half-marathon debacle, the Tesla has been equipped with lasers that shine green lines onto the track, delineating an arrow-shaped wedge that follows six meters behind the car to show the pacers exactly where to run. There are thirty pacers here, all among the best runners in the world, and they've been rehearsing their formation and transitions all week. At the conclusion of each 1.5-mile lap, three of the six pacers drift wide and three fresh pacers merge in from either side of the arrowhead. With Kipchoge, Tadese, and Desisa tucked impassively and unchangingly behind, the pacers and their changeovers, undertaken at high speed and with the very real risk of a catastrophic trip, start to feel like the main attraction. It's like watching a delightfully hypnotic, if somewhat minimalist, ballet.

But change comes soon enough—far sooner than anyone had hoped. After just ten miles, Desisa once again begins to drift off the back of the pack; then, before halfway, Tadese also drops off. In an all-out race against the clock like this, there's virtually no chance that either of them will be able to rally. Whatever magic Nike has tried to conjure suddenly seems awfully thin; it will be Kipchoge or no one, with the latter option looking more and more likely. I've read a raft of articles in recent weeks explaining why the two-hour goal is ludicrous and how spectacularly the runners will pay for their hubris if they try to maintain such a heady pace; I find myself dreading the endless I-told-you-sos that will follow a failure.

But as the pacers and their sole remaining follower pass the halfway point in 59:54, a cheering thought occurs to me. "With every step Kipchoge now takes," I tap into the Twitter app on my phone, "it's the fastest a human has ever run for this distance."

My notebook from the second half of the race is nearly empty. Along with everyone else in the stadium, and millions of people watching live online, I'm fixated on Kipchoge—the blur of his legs, the absence of tension in his cheeks, the preternatural calm of his gaze. At first we're simply hoping that he can hang in there long enough to make it respectable. But as laps go by and the clock ticks on, there's a palpable realization that we're witnessing something special—that however it ends, Kipchoge is blowing past almost everyone's expectations of what humans are capable of. After about ninety minutes, I find Marcora in the throng crowded alongside the finish line. He arches his eyebrows in amazement; I arch mine in return, and we both turn back to the track in silence. There's nothing more to say.

It's during my guest spot in the broadcasting booth that I finally permit myself to think, *Yes. Maybe he really can.*

By the time I sprint though the maze of corridors and down the stairs to the track, there are exactly two 1.5-mile laps remaining—and, almost imperceptibly, Kipchoge has finally begun to falter. There's a tightness in his face, and what looked like occasional smiles are now revealed to be grimaces. The pacers' tight arrowhead is starting to un-ravel as they have to decide between sticking with the Tesla on two-hour pace, or dropping back to continue blocking wind for Kipchoge, who has fallen a little more than ten seconds behind his goal pace.

The greatest endurance athletes in the world, I remind myself, share a trait with the eleven-year-olds in Dominic Micklewright's pacing studies: they always have a finishing kick. Kipchoge's legs are getting heavier, the tide of metabolites in his muscles is rising, his fuel stores are waning—in countless ways, his body is telling him that he has reached his limit and can no longer sustain this pace. But is his brain harboring a final reserve that it will unleash when the finish is within reach?

The wheels don't fall off; Kipchoge doesn't hit the wall like Tadese and Desisa, who are now six and fourteen minutes behind, respec-tively. But he doesn't manage to reaccelerate. Fighting all the way to the finish, he crosses the line in 2:00:25, pauses for the briefest of moments, and then jogs on toward his longtime coach, Patrick Sang, who wraps him in a silent embrace. Then, gingerly, he lowers himself to the ground, lies back, and covers his eyes. All around me, people are hugging, high-fiving, and screaming with raw emotion. While Kipchoge didn't run sub-two, and thanks to the pacing arrangement didn't set an official world record, I have no doubt that I've witnessed a watershed moment in the pursuit of human limits. Future marathon times will *sound* different in light of what just happened.

Over the weeks that follow, there will be endless debate about the keys behind Kipchoge's breakthrough. How much, if at all, did the new shoes help him? What about the experimental Swedish sports drink that encapsulates carbohydrate in a special hydrogel to facilitate absorption, which Kipchoge decided at the last minute to use—did that help him stave off a bonk? And did the Tesla pace car, with its bulky roof-mounted clock, provide a hidden additional drafting aid? "What was the secret, they wanted to know," John L. Parker Jr.'s miler hero laments in *Once a Runner;* "in a thousand different ways they wanted to know *The Secret.*"

Even Nike can't answer these questions—not so much because the answers are confidential (which they are) but because they're all but unknowable. At a conference in Denver a few weeks later, University of Colorado researchers Wouter Hoogkamer and Rodger Kram present the results of their external testing of the Vaporfly shoe. It really does improve running economy by an average of 4 percent. Clearly that doesn't translate directly to 4 percent faster in a marathon, unless you believe Kipchoge in normal shoes is just a 2:05 guy, but scientists offer widely varying opinions about how big the real-world edge is. My back-of-the-envelope triangulation is that they were worth about a minute to Kipchoge—and that includes the mental edge he gained from knowing he was wearing the fastest shoes ever tested.

In the immediate aftermath of the race, though, the question that sticks in my mind is the opposite: How much *faster* could Kipchoge have gone if he'd had a rival with him in those final two laps? We know, after all, that racing against even virtual competition can boost performance by a percent or two compared to time-trialing against the clock. In a head-to-head race, could he have summoned the finishing kick that is nearly always seen in world-record runs? On reflection, though, I conclude that this is unlikely. The peculiar circumstances of the Nike race—the predetermined pace, the tiny field, the absence of any sort of tactical considerations—allowed Kipchoge to fully extend himself. With no rivals to fear, he was able to leave his throat exposed and simply run until his legs could no longer carry him. The half-marathon in March, he had claimed, was just 60 percent effort; that wasn't the case here.

"Today was one hundred percent," he confirms, smiling, a few minutes after finishing. "But you know, we are human."

It's precisely that fact—his very human vulnerability—that has made Kipchoge's run such gripping viewing for everyone who stayed up late or stumbled out of bed to watch it. And it's what connects all of us, as we confront our own personal limits on the bike paths and mountain trails of the world, to those pushing back the limits of our species. Nothing is inevitable; nothing is simply mathematical. Kipchoge, I decide, has just come as close as anyone to truly touching the outer perimeters of his physical capacity. And that leaves me excited about the future—because, as he insists amid the good-natured post-race tumult on the racetrack in Monza, it was never just about him. "The *world* now," he says, "is just twenty-five seconds away."

Acknowledgments

At the heart of this book are the scientists whose work it explores. I'm deeply grateful to all those—too numerous to list individually, though many of their names appear in the preceding pages—who returned my emails, sat through repeated phone calls, and in some cases welcomed me into their labs. Ross Tucker shared raw data for the graph in Chapter 3 with me. Tim Noakes, Samuele Marcora, Alexis Mauger, Guillaume Millet, Stephen Cheung, John Hawley, Lori Haase, Martin Paulus, Kai Lutz, Rodger Kram, and especially Mark Burnley read portions of the manuscript for accuracy. The errors that remain are mine alone, but there would have been far more without their help.

It's thanks to the guidance and patience of my literary agent, Rick Broadhead, and Peter Hubbard of William Morrow that this is an actual book rather than a really long and unreadable blog post. I'm also grateful to the magazine editors who underwrote my book reporting by assigning me stories, in particular Christine Fennessy, Jeremy Keehn, Anthony Lydgate, and Scott Rosenfield. As a result of these assignments, some of the reporting in this book has previously appeared in *Runner's World, Outside, The New Yorker,* the *Walrus,* and the *Globe and Mail.* In the vast majority of cases, this material has substantially changed, but there are a few places where the original sentences I wrote were still the best description or explanation I could come up with.

Cindy Slater of the H. J. Lutcher Stark Center for Physical Culture & Sports, at the University of Texas at Austin, tracked down an obscure Soviet-era study for me, and Gennady Sheyner graciously translated it from Russian for me. My uncle, Wolf Rasmussen, provided over-the-phone translation of nineteenth-century German journals. Flora Tsui coaxed an excellent author photo out of me (if I do say so myself).

Acknowledgments

My thinking about endurance (and just about everything else) has been shaped by ongoing conversations with many peers and mentors, both within journalism and beyond it. I'd like to particularly thank Amby Burfoot, Michael Joyner, David Epstein, Christie Aschwanden, Steve Magness, Brad Stulberg, Jonathan Wai, Terry Laughlin, and Scott Douglas. I might have finished the book more quickly without the distraction of your conversation, but it would have been a lesser book!

Finally, and most important of all, I couldn't have written this book without my family. My parents, Moira and Roger, offered indefatigable research help and extra childcare; on a more fundamental level, their immeasurable and ongoing support throughout my life is what has allowed me to pursue a career as a writer. And to my wife and closest friend, Lauren, and our children, Ella and Natalie: Thank you for everything and I love you.

Notes

TWO HOURS: MAY 6, 2017

1 *an estimated 13 million people*: Take all audience estimates with a grain of salt, but 13.1 million is Nike's official tally of viewers tuned into the live stream on Twitter, Facebook, and YouTube during the race. Another 6.7 million watched the video over the following week, and that number doesn't include China, where a substantial (but untracked) audience watched.

2 *What would happen, Joyner wondered*: "Modeling: Optimal Marathon Performance on the Basis of Physiological Factors," *Journal of Applied Physiology* 70, no. 2 (1991).

2 *"A lot of people scratched their heads"*: This and other details are from multiple conversations with Joyner, but he repeats this quote here: Michael Joyner, "Believe It: A Sub-2 Marathon Is Coming," Runnersworld.com, May 6, 2017.

3 *published an updated paper*: Michael Joyner et al., "The Two-Hour Marathon: Who and When?," *Journal of Applied Physiology* 110 (2011): 275–77; the thirty-eight responses followed in the same issue.

3 *Runner's World magazine asked me*: "What Will It Take to Run a 2-Hour Marathon?," *Runner's World*, November 2014.

3 *biggest sports brand in the world*: The Forbes Fab 40 pegs Nike's brand value at $15 billion, well ahead of ESPN in second place.

CHAPTER 1: THE UNFORGIVING MINUTE

7 *If you can fill the unforgiving minute*: From the poem "If—," by Rudyard Kipling, in *Rewards and Fairies* (London: Macmillan, 1910).

7 *the quintessential "nearly man."*: Sebastian Coe, "Landy the Nearly Man," *Telegraph*, January 26, 2004.

7 *"four-minute mile is beyond my capabilities"*: As quoted in Neal Bascomb, *The Perfect Mile* (London: CollinsWillow, 2004). This definitive account is also the source of subsequent details about Landy's races.

9 *Ernest Shackleton's ill-fated Antarctic expedition*: Alfred Lansing, *Endurance* (New York: Basic Books, 1959).

10 *"the struggle to continue against a mounting desire to stop."*: Marcora cites this as the definition of an "effortful cognitive process," drawing on a definition of stamina from Roy Baumeister et al. in "The Strength Model of Self-Control," *Current Directions in Psychological Science* 16, no. 6 (2007).

10 *LeBron James's biggest foe*: Cork Gaines, "LeBron James Has Played More Minutes Than Anyone in the NBA Since 2010, and It Isn't Even Close," *Business Insider*, June 4, 2015; Tom Withers, "LeBron James Pushes Himself to Total Exhaustion in Win Over

Hawks," Associated Press, May 25, 2015; Chris Mannix, "Do LeBron, Cavaliers Have Enough Left in the Tank to Survive NBA Finals?," *Sports Illustrated,* June 12, 2015.

10 *"Negative Acceleration Phase.":* Jimson Lee, "From the Archives: Maximal Speed and Deceleration," March 17, 2010, and "Usain Bolt 200 Meter Splits, Speed Reserve and Speed Endurance," August 21, 2009, SpeedEndurance.com; Rolf Graubner and Eberhard Nixdorf, "Biomechanical Analysis of the Sprint and Hurdles Events at the 2009 IAAF World Championships in Athletics," *New Studies in Athletics* 1, no. 2 (2011).

10 *Bolt's 9.58-second world-record race:* Bolt's late-race surges can be partly explained by the fact that he reaches a higher top speed, which means that even if his *relative* deceleration in the final 20 meters is the same as everyone else's, he'll continue to pull away. But expert consensus is that he's also uniquely good at late-race "speed maintenance."

11 *Even in repeated all-out weightlifting efforts:* I. Halperin et al., "Pacing Strategies During Repeated Maximal Voluntary Contractions," *European Journal of Applied Physiology* 114, no. 7 (2014).

13 *the prospects of a sub-two-hour marathon:* For the analogy to the four-minute mile, see Claire Dorotik-Nana, "The Four Minute Mile, the Two Hour Marathon, and the Danger of Glass Ceilings," PsychCentral.com, May 5, 2017. For skeptical takes, see Robert Johnson, "The Myth of the Sub-2-Hour Marathon," LetsRun.com, May 6, 2013; and Ross Tucker, "The 2-Hour Marathon and the 4-Min Mile," *Science of Sport,* December 16, 2014.

13 *Spanish star José Luis González became the three hundredth man:* According to the list maintained by the National Union of Track Statisticians, https://nuts.org.uk/sub-4/sub4-dat.htm.

14 *TV coverage of the 1996 Trials is on YouTube:* https://www.youtube.com/watch?v=8d SLUVmK1Ik (but please don't watch it; it wasn't my finest hour).

14 *"It should be mathematical,":* Michael Heald, "It Should Be Mathematical," *Propeller,* Summer 2012.

CHAPTER 2: THE HUMAN MACHINE

17 *After fifty-six days of hard skiing:* Details of Worsley's 2009 expedition and Shackleton's 1909 expedition are from Worsley's 2011 book, *In Shackleton's Footsteps,* unless otherwise noted.

17 *just 112 miles from the South Pole.:* the figure is often reported as "97 miles" because Shackleton (and Worsley) reported their distances in nautical miles, which are about 15 percent longer than the more familiar statute miles. All mile distances in this book are statute unless otherwise noted.

18 *"The decision to turn back,":* From an archived interview broadcast on BBC *Newsnight* on January 26, 2016: https://www.youtube.com/watch?v=O3SMkxA08T8.

18 *between 6,000 and 10,000 calories per day:* Timothy Noakes, "The Limits of Endurance Exercise," *Basic Research in Cardiology* 101 (2006): 408–17. See also Noakes in *Hypoxia and the Circulation,* ed. R. C. Roach et al. (New York: Springer, 2007).

19 *an account of their research on lactic acid:* W. M. Fletcher and F. G. Hopkins, "Lactic Acid in Amphibian Muscle," *Journal of Physiology* 35, no. 4 (1907).

19 *what's found inside the body is actually lactate:* L. B. Gladden, "Lactate Me-

tabolism: A New Paradigm for the Third Millennium," *Journal of Physiology* 558, no. 1 (2004).

19 *Berzelius noticed that the muscles of hunted stags:* This anecdote shows up in many modern textbooks (e.g., *The History of Exercise Physiology,* ed. Charles M. Tipton, 2014) but proved unexpectedly hard to trace. Berzelius first published the observation of lactic acid extracted from the muscles of slaughtered animals in 1808 (in his Swedish book *Föreläsningar i Djurkemien,* p. 176), but many chemists didn't believe it. When the German chemist Justus von Liebig tried to claim credit for the discovery in 1846, Berzelius wrote an indignant response pegging the year of his own observation as 1807 (*Jahresbericht über die Fortschritte der Chemie und Mineralogie,* 1848, p. 586). But Berzelius himself never published the claim that the amount of lactic acid depended on the severity of pre-death exercise. Instead, this observation, attributed to Berzelius, first appears in the 1842 textbook *Lehrbuch der physiologischen Chemie,* by Carl Lehmann, on p. 285. In 1859, the physiologist Emil du Bois-Reymond wrote to Lehmann asking for the source of this statement; Lehmann replied that he had received a personal letter from Berzelius himself reporting that the muscles of hunted animals contained more lactic acid than normal, while animals whose legs were immobilized in splints before death had less lactic acid (reported in *Journal für praktische Chemie,* 1859, p. 240; reprinted in the 1877 book *Gesammelte Abhandlungen zur allgemeinen Muskel- und Nervenphysik* with a footnote describing the exchange of letters on p. 32.).

19 *chemists were still almost a century away:* An oft-cited benchmark in the understanding of acids is Svante Arrhenius's definition, an extension of work that earned him the 1903 Nobel Prize in Chemistry.

19 *Berzelius himself subscribed to the idea of a "vital force":* Berzelius's views on vitalism were actually quite nuanced and evolved over time, as discussed in Bent Søren Jørgensen, "More on Berzelius and the Vital Force," *Journal of Chemical Education* 42, no. 7 (1965).

20 *German scientists collected their own urine:* Dorothy Needham, *Machina Carnis* (Cambridge: Cambridge University Press, 1972).

20 *measure lactate in real time:* Linda Geddes, "Wearable Sweat Sensor Paves Way for Real-Time Analysis of Body Chemistry," *Nature,* January 27, 2016. It's not yet clear, though, how closely lactate levels in sweat correspond to what's happening in your bloodstream or muscles.

20 *first to complete the 320-meter circuit:* Christopher Thorne, "Trinity Great Court Run: The Facts," *Track Stats* 27, no. 3 (1989). There are different schools of thought on the "correct" route around the courtyard, so Fletcher's corner-cutting shouldn't be taken as a mark against his character.

21 *the importance of oxygen was confirmed:* Leonard Hill, "Oxygen And Muscular Exercise as a Form of Treatment," *British Medical Journal* 2, no. 2492 (1908).

22 *He ultimately made twenty-two attempts:* "Jabez Wolffe Dead: English Swimmer, 66," *New York Times,* October 23, 1943.

22 *"[E]very living being has from its birth a limit":* T. S. Clouson, "Female Education from a Medical Point of View," *Popular Science Monthly,* December 1883, p. 215, cited by John Hoberman in *Athletic Enhancement, Human Nature, and Ethics* (New York: Springer, 2013), p. 263.

22 *he hated his name:* William Van der Kloot, "Mirrors and Smoke: A. V. Hill, His Brigands, and the Science of Anti-Aircraft Gunnery in World War I," *Notes & Records of the Royal Society* 65 (2011): 393–410.

23 *In 1923, Hill:* A. V. Hill and Hartley Lupton, "Muscular Exercise, Lactic Acid, and the Supply and Utilization of Oxygen," *Quarterly Journal of Medicine* 16, no. 62 (1923). Details in subsequent paragraphs are also from this paper unless otherwise noted.

23 *"it may well have been my struggles and failures":* A. V. Hill, *Muscular Activity* (Baltimore: Williams & Wilkins, 1925).

23 *an eighty-five-meter grass loop in Hill's garden:* In Hill's 1923 *QMJ* paper, he describes the experiments taking place "around a circular grass track 92½ yds. (84½ metres) in circumference." Hugh Long, a coauthor and experimental subject in Hill's Manchester studies, recalls "running up and down stairs, or round the professor's garden while at intervals healthy samples of blood were withdrawn from my arms"; quoted in "Archibald Vivian Hill. 26 September 1886–3 June 1977," *Biographical Memoirs of Fellows of the Royal Society* 24 (1978): 71–149.

23 *"reaches a maximum beyond which no effort can drive it":* Hill, *Muscular Activity,* p. 98.

24 *an analysis of world records:* A. V. Hill, "The Physiological Basis of Athletic Records," *Nature,* October 10, 1925. For Hill's ideas on muscle viscosity, see *Muscular Movement in Man* (New York: McGraw-Hill, 1927). For details of the hacksaw blade timing system, see Hill's article "Are Athletes Machines?," *Scientific American,* August 1927.

26 *He rode a Harley, taught needlepoint to prison inmates,:* Stefano Hatfield, "This Is the Side of Antarctic Explorer Henry Worsley That the Media Shies Away From," *Independent,* January 31, 2016.

27 *"As you probably are the first to reach this area":* Edward Evans, *South with Scott* (London: Collins, 1921).

27 *a botched "scientific" calculation:* Lewis Halsey and Mike Stroud, "Could Scott Have Survived with Today's Physiological Knowledge?," *Current Biology* 21, no. 12 (2011).

28 *On November 13, he set off on skis:* Details of Henry Worsley's Shackleton solo trip are from the daily audio dispatches he posted at https://soundcloud.com/shackleton solo (the last five days have been removed). Further background details about his trip are at shackletonsolo.org.

29 *"we don't do it because it is useful . . .":* Hill, *Muscular Movement in Man.*

29 *funded by Britain's Industrial Fatigue Research Board:* See author notes in A. V. Hill, C.N.H. Long, and H. Lupton, "Muscular Exercise, Lactic Acid, and the Supply and Utilization of Oxygen," *Proceedings of the Royal Society B* 96 (1924): 438–75.

29 *established in 1927:* Charles Tipton, ed., *History of Exercise Physiology* (Champaign, IL: Human Kinetics, 2014).

29 *Citing Hill's research as his inspiration:* David Bassett Jr., "Scientific Contributions of A. V. Hill: Exercise Physiology Pioneer," *Journal of Applied Physiology* 93, no. 5 (2002).

30 *blood sugar levels in Harvard football players:* Alison Wrynn, "The Athlete in the Making: The Scientific Study of American Athletic Performance, 1920–1932," *Sport in History* 30, no. 1 (2010).

30 *"New Records in Human Power":* S. Robinson et al., "New Records in Human Power," *Science* 85, no. 2208 (1937).

30 *As MIT historian Robin Scheffler recounts:* "The Power of Exercise and the Exercise of Power: The Harvard Fatigue Laboratory, Distance Running, and the Disappearance of Work, 1919–1947," *Journal of the History of Biology* 48 (2015): 391–423.

30 *thirteen workers died of heat exhaustion:* A. D. Hopkins, "Hoover Dam: The Legend Builders," *Nevada*, May/June 1985; Andrew Dunbar and Dennis McBride, *Building Hoover Dam: An Oral History of the Great Depression* (Las Vegas: University of Nevada Press, 2001).

31 *The most notorious of these wartime studies:* Todd Tucker, *The Great Starvation Experiment* (Minneapolis: University of Minnesota Press, 2006).

32 *"there is good reason for not trusting the subject's . . .":* Henry Longstreet Taylor et al., "Maximal Oxygen Intake as an Objective Measure of Cardio-Respiratory Performance," *Journal of Applied Physiology* 8, no. 1 (1955).

32 *"men must have certain minimum physiological requirements":* W. P. Leary and C. H. Wyndham, "The Capacity for Maximum Physical Effort of Caucasian and Bantu Athletes of International Class," *South African Medical Journal* 39, no. 29 (1965).

32 *". . . more in athletics than sheer chemistry,":* Hill, *Muscular Movement in Man.*

32 *"those qualities of resolution . . .":* A. V. Hill, C.N.H. Long, and H. Lupton, "Muscular Exercise, Lactic Acid, and the Supply and Utilization of Oxygen—Parts IV–VI," *Proceedings of the Royal Society B* 97 (1924): 84–138.

33 *on the verge of dropping out:* From interviews with Michael Joyner; see also Ed Caesar, *Two Hours* (New York: Penguin, 2015).

35 *what pushed him over the edge:* Worsley's widow, Joanna Worsley, has suggested that a burst ulcer triggered the infection that killed him: Tom Rowley, "Explorer Henry Worsley's Widow Plans Antarctic Voyage to Say a 'Final Goodbye,'" *Telegraph*, January 7, 2017.

36 *"did Worsley not realize . . .":* Jill Homer, "Henry Worsley and the Psychology of Endurance in Life or Death Situations," *Guardian*, January 26, 2016.

36 *"The machinery of the body . . .":* Hill, *Muscular Movement in Man.*

36 *"I said, now hold on . . .":* Quotes are from my visit to Noakes's lab in Cape Town in 2010.

CHAPTER 3: THE CENTRAL GOVERNOR

37 *Diane Van Deren needed to cover 36 miles:* The Mountains-to-Sea Trail run is recounted in Mackenzie Lobby Havey, "Running from the Seizures," *Atlantic*, December 12, 2014; and Chris Gragtmans, "Diane Van Deren's Record-Setting MST Run," *Blue Ridge Outdoors.* Her background story is told in Bill Donahue, "Fixing Diane's Brain," *Runner's World*, February 2011; John Branch, "Brain Surgery Frees Runner, but Raises Barriers," *New York Times*, July 8, 2009; Hoda Kotb, *Ten Years Later* (New York: Simon & Schuster, 2013).

39 *Noakes started out as a collegiate rower:* most biographical details are from my interviews with him, with additional information from his 2012 memoir (with Michael Vlismas), *Challenging Beliefs.*

39 *gathering of sports scientists before the 1976 New York Marathon:* "The Marathon: Physiological, Medical, Epidemiological, and Psychological Studies," whose proceedings were published in volume 301 of the *Annals of the New York Academy of Sciences* in 1977.

39 *the case of Elanor Sadler:* Noakes's initial report, "Comrades Makes Medical History—Again," appeared in *SA Runner* in September 1981. The case first appeared in a scientific journal in 1985: T. D. Noakes et al., "Water Intoxication: A Possible Complication During Endurance Exercise," *Medicine & Science in Sports & Exercise* 17, no. 3 (1985).

40 *a handful of deaths:* An exact count of deaths due to hyponatremia during endurance exercise is hard to pin down, but one 2007 study tallied eight confirmed and four suspected cases: Mitchell Rosner and Justin Kirven, "Exercise-Associated Hyponatremia," *Clinical Journal of the American Society of Nephrology* 2, no. 1 (2007).

40 *the limits might reside in the contractility:* T. D. Noakes, "Implications of Exercise Testing for Prediction of Athletic Performance: A Contemporary Perspective," *Medicine & Science in Sports & Exercise* 20, no. 4 (1988).

40 Lore of Running, *a 944-page doorstopper:* The book has gone through many editions. The fourth edition, published in 2002, has 944 pages.

40 *the J. B. Wolffe Memorial Lecture:* "Challenging Beliefs: Ex Africa Semper Aliquid Novi," *Medicine & Science in Sports & Exercise* 29, no. 5 (1997).

41 *Gage was "no longer Gage.":* "Recovery from the Passage of an Iron Bar through the Head," *Publications of the Massachusetts Medical Society* 2, no. 3 (1868).

42 *"You must have just come through those tornadoes back there,":* Quoted in Havey, "Running from the Seizures."

42 *"is the hardest thing I have ever done.":* Quoted in "900+ Miles Later, Diane Van Deren Reaches Jockey's Ridge," greatoutdoorprovision.com, 2012.

43 *"Well, shit—I don't feel pain?":* Quoted in Kotb, *Ten Years Later.*

43 *"I could be out running for two weeks,":* Quoted in Andrea Minarcek, "Going the Distance," *National Geographic,* December 2009/January 2010.

43 *largest, oldest, and most prestigious ultra-race:* First run in 1921, Comrades earned a place in the Guinness record books in 2010 with 16,480 starters and 14,343 finishers within the twelve-hour time limit. In 2000, prior to Guinness certification, more than 20,000 people finished, according to the official results at www.comrades.com.

45 *in a 1998 paper he coined the term "central governor,":* In "Maximal Oxygen Uptake: 'Classical' versus 'Contemporary' Viewpoints: A Rebuttal," *Medicine & Science in Sports & Exercise* 30, no. 9 (1998), Noakes writes: "a new physiological model is proposed in which skeletal muscle recruitment is regulated by a central 'governor' specifically to prevent the development of a progressive myocardial ischemia that would precede the development of skeletal muscle anaerobiosis during maximum exercise."

45 *Alan St. Clair Gibson:* See, for example, T. D. Noakes, A. St. Clair Gibson, and E. V. Lambert, "From Catastrophe to Complexity: A Novel Model of Integrative Central Neural Regulation of Effort and Fatigue During Exercise in Humans," *British Journal of Sports Medicine* 38, no. 4 (2004).

45 *Frank Marino:* See, for example, "Anticipatory Regulation and Avoidance of Catastrophe During Exercise-Induced Hyperthermia," *Comparative Biochemistry and Physiology–Part B* 139, no. 4 (2004).

46 *a critical threshold of about 104 degrees Fahrenheit:* B. Nielsen et al., "Human Circulatory and Thermoregulatory Adaptations with Heat Acclimation and Exercise in a Hot, Dry Environment," *Journal of Physiology* 460 (1993): 467–85; J. González-Alonso et al., "Influence of Body Temperature on the Development of Fatigue During Prolonged Exercise in the Heat," *Journal of Applied Physiology* 86, no. 3 (1999).

46 *cyclists started at a slower pace:* R. Tucker et al., "Impaired Exercise Performance in the Heat Is Associated with an Anticipatory Reduction in Skeletal Muscle Recruitment," *Pflügers Archiv* 448, no. 4 (2004).

46 *puzzlingly low lactate levels:* T. D. Noakes, "Evidence That Reduced Skeletal Muscle Recruitment Explains the Lactate Paradox During Exercise at High Altitude," *Journal of Applied Physiology* 106 (2009): 737–38.

46 *swish a carbohydrate drink:* J. M. Carter et al., "The Effect of Carbohydrate Mouth Rinse on 1-h Cycle Time Trial Performance," *Medicine & Science in Sports & Exercise* 36, no. 12 (2004).

46 *supposedly crippling levels of dehydration:* Lukas Beis et al., "Drinking Behaviors of Elite Male Runners During Marathon Competition," *Clinical Journal of Sports Medicine* 22, no. 3.

46 *brain-altering drugs like Tylenol:* A. R. Mauger et al., "Influence of Acetaminophen on Performance During Time Trial Cycling," *Journal of Applied Physiology* 108, no. 1 (2010).

48 *pacing patterns of almost every world record:* R. Tucker et al., "An Analysis of Pacing Strategies During Men's World-Record Performances in Track Athletics," *International Journal of Sports Physiology and Performance* 1, no. 3 (2006).

49 *"If they caught you breaching, . . .":* This and other details from Micklewright's talk at the Endurance Research Conference at the University of Kent in September 2015.

49 *Micklewright had more than a hundred schoolchildren:* D. Micklewright et al., "Pacing Strategy in Schoolchildren Differs with Age and Cognitive Development," *Medicine & Science in Sports & Exercise* 44, no. 2 (2012).

50 *finish times of more than nine million marathoners:* Eric Allen et al., "Reference-Dependent Preferences: Evidence from Marathon Runners," *Management Science* 63, no. 6 (2016).

51 *"produced a brainless model of human exercise performance.":* T. D. Noakes, "Testing for Maximum Oxygen Consumption Has Produced a Brainless Model of Human Exercise Performance," *British Journal of Sports Medicine* 42, no. 7 (2008).

51 *"In the parlance of my North American colleagues,":* Roy Shephard, "The Author's Reply," *Sports Medicine* 40, no. 1 (2010).

52 *a disciplinary hearing:* Bill Gifford, "The Silencing of a Low-Carb Rebel," *Outside,* December 8, 2016.

52 *video of a Rube Goldberg-esque contraption:* https://www.youtube.com/watch?v=L8SghDfyo-8; E. B. Fontes et al., "Brain Activity and Perceived Exertion During Cycling Exercise: An fMRI Study," *British Journal of Sports Medicine* 49, no. 8 (2015).

52 *Other researchers have tried electroencephalography:* L. Hilty et al., "Fatigue-Induced Increase in Intracortical Communication Between Mid/Anterior Insular and Motor Cortex During Cycling Exercise," *European Journal of Neuroscience* 34, no. 12 (2011).

CHAPTER 4: THE CONSCIOUS QUITTER

55 *Marcora's thirteen-thousand-mile motorcycle ride:* To hear Marcora himself spinning tales from this trip, check out his podcast appearance on the Adventure Rider Radio Motorcycle Podcast from May 15, 2015, https://adventureriderpodcast.libsyn.com/.

57 *I drove 120 miles through Australia's Blue Mountains:* I wrote about this trip

and my subsequent experience with Marcora's brain endurance training in the October 2013 issue of *Runner's World.*

57 *among the* New York Times–*reading public:* Nicholas Bakalar, "Behavior: Mental Fatigue Can Lead to Physical Kind," *New York Times,* March 9, 2009. The study was S. M. Marcora et al., "Mental Fatigue Impairs Physical Performance in Humans," *Journal of Applied Physiology* 106, no. 3 (2009).

58 *". . . the single best indicator of the degree of physical strain,":* Gunnar Borg, "Psychophysical Bases of Perceived Exertion," *Medicine & Science in Sports & Exercise* 14, no. 5 (1982).

60 *a 1986 experiment by French researcher Michel Cabanac:* "Money Versus Pain: Experimental Study of a Conflict in Humans," *Journal of the Experimental Analysis of Behavior* 46, no. 1 (1986).

60 *a similar mind-over-muscle demonstration:* S. M. Marcora and W. Staiano, "The Limits to Exercise Tolerance in Humans: Mind over Muscle?," *European Journal of Applied Physiology* 109, no. 4 (2010).

61 *a bewilderingly complex slide taken from a recent paper:* Chris Abbiss and Paul Laursen, "Models to Explain Fatigue During Prolonged Cycling," *Sports Medicine* 35, no. 10 (2005).

62 *Angelo Mosso conducted a series of experiments:* A 1904 translation of *La Fatica* is available at https://archive.org/details/fatigue01drumgoog. For further context, see Camillo Di Giulio et al., "Angelo Mosso and Muscular Fatigue: 116 years After the First Congress of Physiologists: IUPS Commemoration," *Advances in Physiology Education* 30, no. 2 (2006).

63 *Mosso's insights were mostly forgotten:* Tim Noakes argues that Mosso's ideas were supplanted by those of A. V. Hill: "Fatigue Is a Brain-Derived Emotion That Regulates the Exercise Behavior to Ensure the Protection of Whole Body Homeostasis," *Frontiers in Physiology,* April 11, 2012.

63 *The torch passed instead to psychologists:* Nick Joyce and David Baker, "The Early Days of Sports Psychology," *Monitor on Psychology,* July/August 2008.

63 *An 1898 study by Indiana University psychologist Norman Triplett:* "The Dynamogenic Factors in Pacemaking and Competition," *American Journal of Psychology* 9, no. 4 (1898).

64 *a famous 1988 experiment:* Fritz Strack et al., "Inhibiting and Facilitating Conditions of the Human Smile: A Nonobtrusive Test of the Facial Feedback Hypothesis," *Journal of Personality and Social Psychology* 54, no. 5 (1988).

64 *record the activity of facial muscles:* H. M. de Morree and S. M. Marcora, "The Face of Effort: Frowning Muscle Activity Reflects Effort During a Physical Task," *Biological Psychology* 85, no. 3 (2010), and "Frowning Muscle Activity and Perception of Effort During Constant-Workload Cycling," *European Journal of Applied Psychology* 112, no. 5 (2012).

64 *subsequent study by Taiwanese researchers:* D. H. Huang et al., "Frowning and Jaw Clenching Muscle Activity Reflects the Perception of Effort During Incremental Workload Cycling," *Journal of Sports Science and Medicine* 13, no. 4 (2014).

64 *legendary sprint coach Bud Winter:* Tex Maule, "It's Agony, Upsets and Hopes," *Sports Illustrated,* June 15, 1959.

65 *cyclists who were shown sad faces rode:* A. Blanchfield et al., "Non-Conscious Visual Cues Related to Affect and Action Alter Perception of Effort and Endurance Performance," *Frontiers in Human Neuroscience,* December 11, 2014.

65 *tested a simple self-talk intervention:* A. Blanchfield et al., "Talking Yourself Out of Exhaustion: The Effects of Self-Talk on Endurance Performance," *Medicine & Science in Sports & Exercise* 46, no. 5 (2014).

66 *caffeine pills:* F. C. Wardenaar et al., "Nutritional Supplement Use by Dutch Elite and Sub-Elite Athletes: Does Receiving Dietary Counseling Make a Difference?," *International Journal of Sport Nutrition and Exercise Metabolism* 2, no. 1 (2017).

67 *his famous "marshmallow test":* Walter Mischel et al., "Delay of Gratification in Children," *Science* 244, no. 4907 (1989); also B. J. Casey et al., "Behavioral and Neural Correlates of Delay of Gratification 40 Years Later," *PNAS* 108, no. 36 (2011).

68 *tax their subjects' response inhibition:* B. Pageaux et al., "Response Inhibition Impairs Subsequent Self-Paced Endurance Performance," *European Journal of Applied Physiology* 114, no. 5 (2014).

69 *professionals were significantly better at the Stroop task:* K. Martin et al., "Superior Inhibitory Control and Resistance to Mental Fatigue in Professional Road Cyclists," *PLoS One* 11, no. 7 (2016).

TWO HOURS: NOVEMBER 30, 2016

73 *ushered through security into the Nike Sport Research Lab:* My full account of the build-up to Nike's Breaking2 race, "Moonshot," was published in the June 2017 issue of *Runner's World.* Further commentary and reporting is collected at www.runnersworld .com/2-hour-marathon.

74 *tests secretly conducted at the University of Colorado:* The study was performed in Rodger Kram's group: Wouter Hoogkamer et al., "New Running Shoe Reduces the Energetic Cost of Running," presented at the American College of Sports Medicine annual meeting in Denver, May 31, 2017.

75 *100 seconds over the course of a two-hour marathon:* C. T. Davies, "Effects of Wind Assistance and Resistance on the Forward Motion of a Runner," *Journal of Applied Physiology* 48, no. 4 (1980).

75 *running directly behind another runner can eliminate:* L.G.C.E. Pugh, "The Influence of Wind Resistance in Running and Walking and the Mechanical Efficiency of Work Against Horizontal or Vertical Forces," *Journal of Physiology* 213 (1971): 255–76.

77 *Shalane Flanagan, the second-fastest women's marathoner:* David Epstein noted Flanagan and Hall's early exposure to high altitude in *The Sports Gene* (New York: Current, 2013).

78 *aid tables every five kilometers:* the IAAF Road Running Manual (www.iaaf.org) says "water shall be available at suitable intervals of approximately 5km."

CHAPTER 5: PAIN

83 *the very first stage of the 2014 Tour de France:* Kenny Pryde, "Marcel Kittel Wins Opening Stage of Tour de France," *Cycling Weekly,* July 5, 2014; Mike Fogarty, "'Now I Am Officially the Biggest Climber in the Tour de France'—Jens Voigt," firstendurance .com, July 6, 2014.

83 *coined when a Danish television reporter:* "The Origin of 'Shut Up, Legs!'," *Bicycling,* http://www.bicycling.com/video/origin-shut-legs.

84 *"... pain as a state of mind to be combated ..."*: "Jens Voigt: The Man Behind the Hour Attempt," *Cycling Weekly,* September 17, 2014.

84 *Freund published a telling study:* Wolfgang Freund et al., "Ultra-Marathon Runners Are Different: Investigations into Pain Tolerance and Personality Traits of Participants of the TransEurope FootRace 2009," *Pain Practice* 13, no. 7 (2013).

85 *"The beauty of it lies in its simplicity,"*: from Jens Voigt, *Shut Up, Legs!* (London: Ebury Press, 2016).

85 *The first official Hour record:* Michael Hutchinson, "Hour Record: The Tangled History of an Iconic Feat," *Cycling Weekly,* April 15, 2015. See also Michael Hutchinson, *The Hour* (London: Yellow Jersey, 2006), which recounts his own crack at the record.

86 *The most iconic record of all:* Owen Mulholland, "Eddy and the Hour," *Bicycle Guide,* March 1991; William Fotheringham, *Merckx: Half Man, Half Bike* (Chicago: Chicago Review Press, 2012); Patrick Brady, "The Greatest Season Ever," *Peloton,* February/March 2011.

87 *British journalist and cycling fan Simon Usborne:* Simon Usborne, "As Sir Bradley Wiggins Attempts to Smash the Hour Record—Our Man Takes On the World's Toughest Track Challenge," *Independent,* May 30, 2015.

87 *Among the first to study pain perception in athletes:* Vivien Scott and Karel Gijsbers, "Pain Perception in Competitive Swimmers," *British Medical Journal* 283 (1981): 91–93.

88 *Martyn Morris and Thomas O'Leary:* Martyn Morris et al., "Learning to Suffer: High- But Not Moderate-intensity Training Increases Pain Tolerance: Results from a Randomised Study," presented at the American College of Sports Medicine annual meeting in Denver, June 2, 2017.

89 *"When I'm hurting like crazy,"*: Jesse Thomas, "Damage Control," *Triathlete,* August 12, 2015.

90 *plain old Tylenol:* A. R. Mauger et al., "Influence of Acetaminophen on Performance During Time Trial Cycling," *Journal of Applied Physiology* 108, no. 1 (2010).

91 *"Yes, whenever it was necessary."*: Quoted in *The Economics of Professional Road Cycling,* ed. Daam Van Reeth and Daniel Joseph Larson (Cham: Springer International, 2016).

91 *Frenchman Roger Rivière:* Various versions of Rivière's tale circulate; see, for example, Nick Brownlee, *Vive le Tour! Amazing Tales of the Tour de France* (London: Portico, 2010).

91 *injected the nerve blocker fentanyl:* M. Amann et al., "Opioid-Mediated Muscle Afferents Inhibit Central Motor Drive and Limit Peripheral Muscle Fatigue Development in Humans," *Journal of Physiology* 587, no. 1 (2009).

92 *took to the online journal* Frontiers in Physiology: "Fatigue is a pain—the use of novel neurophysiological techniques to understand the fatigue-pain relationship" (May 13, 2013).

93 *transcutaneous electric nerve stimulation (TENS), and interferential current (IFC):* A. H. Astokorki et al., "Transcutaneous Electrical Nerve Stimulation Reduces Exercise-Induced Perceived Pain and Improves Endurance Exercise Performance," *European Journal of Applied Physiology* 117, no. 3 (2017); A. H. Astokorki et al., "An Investigation into the Analgesic Effects of Transcutaneous Electrical Nerve Stimulation and

Interferential Current on Exercise-Induced Pain and Performance," presented at Endurance Research Conference 2015 at the University of Kent.

93 *the primacy of effort:* W. Staiano et al., "The Sensory Limit to Exercise Tolerance: Pain or Effort?" presented at Endurance Research Conference 2015 at the University of Kent.

94 *Mauger and Marcora teamed up:* L. Angius et al., "The Effect of Transcranial Direct Current Stimulation of the Motor Cortex on Exercise-Induced Pain," *European Journal of Applied Physiology* 115, no. 11 (2015).

96 *Slovenian cross-country skier Petra Majdič:* David Epstein, "The Truth About Pain: It's in Your Head," *Sports Illustrated,* August 8, 2011.

96 *wounded soldiers during the U.S. Civil War:* Silas Weir Mitchell treated soldiers at a special hospital for "stumps and nervous diseases" and made important observations about phantom limb syndrome and nerve-related pain. See, for example, his American Physiological Society biography at http://www.the-aps.org/fm/presidents/SWMitchell .html.

CHAPTER 6: MUSCLE

101 *On a warm Tucson evening:* Alexis Huicochea, "Man Lifts Car off Pinned Cyclist," *Arizona Daily Star,* July 28, 2006; further details in Jeff Wise, *Extreme Fear: The Science of Your Mind in Danger* (New York: Palgrave Macmillan, 2009).

102 *measurement techniques weren't advanced enough:* For a historical review, see S. C. Gandevia, "Spinal and Supraspinal Factors in Human Muscle Fatigue," *Physiological Reviews* 81, no. 4 (2001).

102 *"the end point of any performance . . .":* Michio Ikai and Arthur Steinhaus, "Some Factors Modifying the Expression of Human Strength," *Journal of Applied Physiology* 16, no. 1 (1961).

102 *They piloted Pervitin:* Fabienne Hurst, "The German Granddaddy of Crystal Meth," *Der Spiegel,* May 30, 2013; Andreas Ulrich, "Hitler's Drugged Soldiers," *Der Spiegel,* May 6, 2005.

104 *Israel Halperin at Memorial University:* I. Halperin et al., "Pacing Strategies During Repeated Maximal Voluntary Contractions," *European Journal of Applied Physiology* 114, no. 7 (2014).

105 *"to fill an awful lot of mousetraps.":* You can (and should) watch the 1983 World's Strongest Man competition on YouTube: https://www.youtube.com/watch?v= u8DECs72W4E.

105 *records using standard bars and plates:* There are many different record standards, depending on the use of equipment like lifting straps, to none of which Magee's cheese lift conformed. The current International Powerlifting Federation record is 397.5 kg (876 pounds); Englishman Eddie Hall lifted 500 kg (1,102 pounds) at the World Deadlift Championships in 2016 before collapsing with burst blood vessels in his head.

105 *weighs at least 3,000 pounds:* The first Camaro, in 1967, weighed 2,920 pounds; by 2010, curb weight had ballooned to 3,737 pounds. Murilee Martin, "Model Bloat: How the Camaro Gained 827 Pounds Over 37 Model Years," *Jalopnik,* January 28, 2009.

105 *according to one of Zatsiorsky's studies:* V. M. Zatsiorsky, "Intensity of Strength Training Facts and Theory: Russian and Eastern European Approach," *National Strength and Conditioning Association Journal* 14, no. 5 (1992).

106 *as a pair of Danish researchers wrote:* T. E. Hansen and J. Lindhard, "On the Maximum Work of Human Muscles Especially the Flexors of the Elbow," *Journal of Physiology* 57, no. 5 (1923).

106 *a cheerfully eccentric British physiologist named Patrick Merton:* P. A. Merton, "Voluntary Strength and Fatigue," *Journal of Physiology* 123, no. 3 (1954); Alan J. McComas, "The Neuromuscular System," in *Exercise Physiology: People and Ideas*, ed. Charles Tipton (Oxford and New York: Oxford University Press, 2003); John Rothwell and Ian Glynn, "Patrick Anthony Merton. 8 October 1920–13 June 2: Elected FRS 1979," *Biographical Memoirs of Fellows of the Royal Society* 52 (2006): 189–201.

109 *By the time Stéphane Couleaud:* Couleaud's misadventures at the Tor des Géants are recounted on his blog, stephanecouleaud.blogspot.com: "Tor de Geants 2001–Edizione 2–11/14 sept," October 4, 2011. Some of Couleaud's data is presented in Guillaume Millet's presentation, "Fatigue and Ultra-Endurance Performance," at the Endurance Research Conference at the University of Kent in September 2015, along with Millet's own Tor des Géants experience. The full results of the scientific study are published as Jonas Saugy et al., "Alterations of Neuromuscular Function after the World's Most Challenging Mountain Ultra-Marathon," *PLoS One* 8, no. 6 (2013).

114 *Norwegian researcher Christian Frøyd:* C. Frøyd et al., "Central Regulation and Neuromuscular Fatigue During Exercise of Different Durations," *Medicine & Science in Sports & Exercise* 48, no. 6 (2016).

115 *Ross Tucker's analysis of world record pacing:* "Men's 800m: Anyone's Race and a Discussion of 800m Pacing Physiology," *Science of Sport*, August 22, 2008.

116 *events lasting between about one and ten minutes:* Simeon P. Cairns, "Lactic Acid and Exercise Performance," *Sports Medicine* 36, no. 4 (2006). In absolute terms, the highest levels of lactate may actually occur a few minutes after an all-out exercise bout of 30 to 120 seconds; see Matthew Goodwin et al., "Blood Lactate Measurements and Analysis During Exercise: A Guide for Clinicians," *Journal of Diabetes Science and Technology* 1, no. 4 (2007). But from an athlete's perspective, it doesn't really matter what happens after the race is over.

116 *thanks primarily to George Brooks:* Gina Kolata, "Lactic Acid Is Not Muscles' Foe, It's Fuel," *New York Times*, May 16, 2006.

116 *injecting three different metabolites:* K. A. Pollak et al., "Exogenously Applied Muscle Metabolites Synergistically Evoke Sensations of Muscle Fatigue and Pain in Human Subjects," *Experimental Physiology* 99, no. 2 (2014).

118 *David Epstein recounted the ordeal of Rhiannon Hull:* "Distance Runner Rhiannon Hull," *Sports Illustrated*, March 12, 2012.

CHAPTER 7: OXYGEN

119 *William Trubridge took a deep breath:* A video of the record-setting dive, as broadcast on TVNZ, is available at https://www.tvnz.co.nz/one-news/sport/other/full-dive-watch-kiwi-william-trubridge-set-new-free-diving-world-record. See also "Trubridge Breaks World Free Diving Record," *Radio New Zealand*, July 22, 2016.

119 *Two years earlier, in 2014, Trubridge had attempted:* Liam Hyslop, "Kiwi Freediver William Trubridge Fails Record Attempt," Stuff.co.nz, December 3, 2014.

120 *"dodgy nasal spray":* Michele Hewitson, "Michele Hewitson Interview: William Trubridge," *New Zealand Herald*, October 25, 2014; Nicolas Rossier, "One Breath: The Story of William Trubridge," *Huffington Post*, September 6, 2012.

120 *"So I was brought up on the boat,"*: Quoted in *One Breath–The Story of William Trubridge*, a 2012 short film by Nicolas Rossier.

121 *improbable tales of pearl divers:* James Nestor's 2014 book, *Deep: Freediving, Renegade Science, and What the Ocean Tells Us About Ourselves*, offers an excellent overview of the history, physiology, and culture of freediving.

121 *Raimondo Bucher wagered 50,000 lire:* Accounts vary about the details of Bucher's dive; the details here are as reported by Nestor in *Deep*.

122 *He tried for 800 feet:* Stephan Whelan, "Herbert Nitsch Talks About His Fateful Dive and Recovery," DeeperBlue.com, June 6, 2013.

122 *record isn't without controversy:* Christophe Leray, "New World Record Static Apnea (STA)," Freedive-Earth, http://www.freedive-earth.com/blog/new-world-record-static-apnea-sta.

123 *"a spectacle and experimental field . . .":* Stephan Whelan, "Incredible New Guinness World Record—24 Minute O2 Assisted Breath-Hold," DeeperBlue.com, March 3, 2016.

123 *"Mifsud trains like an endurance athlete":* Laura Maurice, "Stéphane Mifsud recordman du monde d'apnée: 'Là où la vie s'arrête,'" *Le Républicain Lorrain*, April 2, 2015; Guillaume Mollaret, "Onze minutes en apnée pour Mifsud, l'homme poisson," *Le Figaro*, June 9, 2009.

123 *physiologist Charles Richet:* Charles Richet, "De la résistance des canard a l'asphyxie," *Journal de physiologie et de pathologie générale* (1899): 641–50.

123 *coining the term 'ectoplasm':* A Dictionary of Hallucinations, Jan Dirk Blom (New York: Springer, 2010).

124 *Master Switch of Life.:* P. F. Scholander, "The Master Switch of Life," *Scientific American* 209 (1963): 92–106.

124 *underwater for more than 45 minutes:* Of the 87 dives observed in one study of Weddell seals, 86 were roughly 45 minutes or shorter and one was—apparently—82 minutes. Michael Castellini et al., "Metabolic Rates of Freely Diving Weddell Seals: Correlations with Oxygen Stores, Swim Velocity and Diving Duration," *Journal of Experimental Biology* 165 (1992): 181–94.

124 *bottom of a water-filled wooden tank:* C. Robert Olsen, "Some Effects of Breath Holding and Apneic Underwater Diving on Cardiac Rhythm in Man," *Journal of Applied Physiology* 17, no. 3 (1962).

124 *Trubridge's pulse drops into the 20s:* He has recorded a pulse of 27 during dryland training, though he hasn't actually measured similar values during dives (personal communication).

124 *sensors appear to be primarily around the nose:* W. Michael Panneton, "The Mammalian Diving Response: An Enigmatic Reflex to Preserve Life?," *Physiology* 28, no. 5 (2013).

124 *organ is basically a natural scuba tank:* Sarah Milton, "Go Ahead, Vent Your Spleen!," *Journal of Experimental Biology* 207 (2004): 390.

124 *Croatian national freediving team:* Darija Baković et al., "Spleen Volume and Blood Flow Response to Repeated Breath-Hold Apneas," *Journal of Applied Physiology* 95, no. 4 (2003).

125 *heart rate begins to plummet just before it dives:* See Panneton, "The Mammalian Diving Response."

127 *One of the first descriptions of altitude illness:* For historical overview of altitude illness, see John West, *High Life: A History of High-Altitude Physiology and Medicine* (New York: Oxford University Press, 1998).

128 *soldier-turned-mountaineer Edward Norton made it to 28,126 feet:* Norton's account is reproduced in *Everest: Expedition to the Ultimate,* Reinhold Messner's 1979 book about his and Habeler's ascent.

129 *"Because it's there.":* "Climbing Mount Everest Is Work for Supermen," *New York Times,* March 18, 1923.

129 *"No one cares for the prospect . . .":* Quoted in Messner, *Everest.*

129 *sixty men and two women:* The exact tally of Everest summits depends on whom you believe. This number includes the three climbers from the 1960 Chinese expedition (whose claims were greeted with widespread skepticism at the time); it doesn't include Mick Burke, who was last seen a few hundred meters from the summit in 1975 but never returned.

130 *"the rate of ascent must approach zero . . .":* Quoted in West, *High Life.*

130 *he and his brother Günther:* Brad Wetzler, "Reinhold Don't Care What You Think," *Outside,* October 2002.

131 *". . . an ascent without oxygen to be certain suicide.":* Raymond A. Sokolov, "The Lonely Victory," *New York Times,* October 7, 1979.

132 *according to the Himalayan Database:* As cited by Alan Arnette, "Everest by the Numbers: 2017 Edition," AlanArnette.com, December 30, 2016.

132 *John West wrote:* "Human Limits for Hypoxia: The Physiological Challenge of Climbing Mt. Everest," *Annals of the New York Academy of Sciences* 889 (2000): 15–27.

133 *the low-altitude control group lives at over 3,000 feet:* For example, Christoph Siebenmann et al., "'Live High-Train Low' Using Normobaric Hypoxia: A Double-Blinded, Placebo-Controlled Study," *Journal of Applied Physiology* 112, no. 1 (2012).

134 *no difference between sea level and Canberra:* C. J. Gore et al., "Increased Arterial Desaturation in Trained Cyclists During Maximal Exercise at 580 m Altitude," *Journal of Applied Physiology* 80, no. 6 (1996).

134 *about 70 percent of male endurance athletes:* K. Constantini et al., "Prevalence of Exercise-Induced Arterial Hypoxemia in Distance Runners at Sea Level," *Medicine & Science in Sports & Exercise* 49, no. 5 (2017).

134 *sustain an average of 85 percent of her VO_2max:* Ben Londeree, "The Use of Laboratory Test Results with Long Distance Runners," *Sports Medicine* 3 (1986): 201–13.

134 *increases in VO_2max aren't necessarily proportional to increases in race performance:* Niels Vollaard et al., "Systematic Analysis of Adaptations in Aerobic Capacity and Submaximal Energy Metabolism Provides a Unique Insight into Determinants of Human Aerobic Performance," *Journal of Applied Physiology* 106, no. 5 (2009).

135 *in a diverse group of people:* "Aerobic Capacity and Fractional Utilisation of Aerobic Capacity in Elite and Non-elite Male and Female Marathon Runners," *European Journal of Applied Physiology and Occupational Physiology* 52, no. 1 (1983).

135 *a manuscript called "New Records in Human Power":* Thomas Haugen et al., *International Journal of Sports Physiology and Performance,* September 5, 2017.

136 *Oskar Svendsen:* Shane Stokes, "If All Goes to Plan, Big Future Predicted for Junior World Champion Oskar Svendsen," Velonation.com, September 25, 2012; Jarle Fredagsvik, "Oskar Svendsen tar pause fra syklingen," Procycling.no, September 18, 2014.

136 *A later study by AIS scientists:* C. J. Gore et al., "Reduced Performance of Male and Female Athletes at 580 m Altitude," *European Journal of Applied Physiology and Occupational Physiology* 75, no. 2 (1997).

136 *a marathon alongside the Dead Sea:* Jeré Longman, "Man vs. Marathon: One Scientist's Quixotic Quest to Propel a Runner Past the Two-Hour Barrier," *New York Times,* May 11, 2016.

136 *research on "cerebral oxygenation":* F. Billaut et al., "Cerebral Oxygenation Decreases but Does Not Impair Performance During Self-Paced, Strenuous Exercise," *Acta Physiologica* 198, no. 4 (2010); J. Santos-Concejero et al., "Maintained Cerebral Oxygenation During Maximal Self-Paced Exercise in Elite Kenyan Runners," *Journal of Applied Physiology* 118, no. 2 (2015).

137 *An ingenious study by Guillaume Millet:* G. Y. Millet et al., "Severe Hypoxia Affects Exercise Performance Independently of Afferent Feedback and Peripheral Fatigue," *Journal of Applied Physiology* 112, no. 8 (2012).

138 *"lactate paradox":* D. B. Dill, *Life, Heat, and Altitude* (Cambridge, MA: Harvard University Press, 1938); West, *High Life;* Sarah W. Tracy, "The Physiology of Extremes: Ancel Keys and the International High Altitude Expedition of 1935," *Bulletin of the History of Medicine* 86 (2012): 627–60.

138 *"possible explanation for this seeming paradox":* "Evidence That Reduced Skeletal Muscle Recruitment Explains the Lactate Paradox During Exercise at High Altitude," *Journal of Applied Physiology* 106 (2009): 737–38.

139 *mountain climbers who don't adapt well:* M. J. MacInnis and M. S. Koehle, "Evidence for and Against Genetic Predispositions to Acute and Chronic Altitude Illnesses," *High Altitude Medicine & Biology* 17, no. 4 (2016).

CHAPTER 8: HEAT

141 *Blame it on the Kentuckiana sun:* Max Gilpin's death and the subsequent trial of Jason Stinson received extensive and sometimes conflicting media coverage. The key sources I relied on in my account: Rodney Daugherty, *Factors Unknown: The Tragedy That Put a Coach and Football on Trial* (Morley, MO: Acclaim Press, 2011); Thomas Lake, "The Boy Who Died of Football," *Sports Illustrated,* December 6, 2010; and the court documents compiled and made available online (http://datacenter.courier-journal.com/documents/stinson/) by the *Louisville Courier-Journal,* whose reporters led coverage of the incident and its aftermath.

141 *"On the line":* As quoted in Lake.

141 *"We're gonna run":* As quoted in Lake.

141 *"Ding, ding, ding":* as quoted in Daugherty.

143 *more than a million boys:* "2009–10 High School Athletics Participation Survey," National Federation of State High School Associations.

143 *invented sous-vide cooking, and introduced the potato:* Joe Schwarcz, *Monkeys, Myths, and Molecules* (Toronto: ECW Press, 2015).

143 *experiments on a professional cyclist named Melvin A. Mode:* Francis Benedict and Edward Cathcart, *Muscular Work: A Metabolic Study with Special Reference to the Efficiency of the Human Body as a Machine* (Washington, DC, 1913).

144 *tragedy investigated by Griffith Pugh:* "Deaths from Exposure on Four Inns Walking Competition, March 14–15, 1964," *Lancet* 283, no. 7344 (1964).

144 *"hiker's hypothermia":* Andrew Young and John Castellani, "Exertional Fatigue and Cold Exposure: Mechanisms of Hiker's Hypothermia," *Applied Physiology, Nutrition, and Metabolism* 32 (2007): 793–98.

144 *250 milliliters (half a pint) of blood:* Nisha Charkoudian, "Skin Blood Flow in Adult Human Thermoregulation: How It Works, When It Does Not, and Why," *Mayo Clinic Proceedings* 78 (2003): 603–12.

144 *heat at a rate of about 100 watts:* For a comprehensive review, see Matthew Cramer and Ollie Jay, "Biophysical Aspects of Human Thermoregulation During Heat Stress," *Autonomic Neuroscience: Basic and Clinical* 196 (2016): 3–13.

145 *protective responses get progressively better:* J. D. Périard et al., "Adaptations and Mechanisms of Human Heat Acclimation: Applications for Competitive Athletes and Sports," *Scandinavian Journal of Medicine and Science in Sports* 25, no. S1 (2015).

145 *known anecdotally for centuries:* For a historical review, see Charles Tipton, *History of Exercise Physiology* (Champaign, IL: Human Kinetics, 2014).

146 *in South African gold mines:* Aldo Dreosti, "The Results of Some Investigations into the Medical Aspect of Deep Mining on the Witwatersrand," *Journal of the Chemical, Metallurgical and Mining Society of South Africa*, November 1935.

147 *Studies during World War II:* Sid Robinson et al., "Rapid Acclimatization to Work in Hot Climates," *American Journal of Physiology* 140 (1943): 168–76.

147 *researchers at Denmark's storied August Krogh Institute :* J. González-Alonso et al., "Influence of Body Temperature on the Development of Fatigue During Prolonged Exercise in the Heat," *Journal of Applied Physiology* 86, no. 3 (1999).

147 *The Australian Olympic team brought ice baths:* Alex Hutchinson, "Faster, Higher, Sneakier," *Walrus,* January 12, 2010.

148 *Tests by Australian sports scientists:* Rodney Siegel et al., "Ice Slurry Ingestion Increases Core Temperature Capacity and Running Time in the Heat," *Medicine & Science in Sports & Exercise* 42, no. 4 (2010).

148 *temperature sensors in your stomach:* N. B. Morris et al., "Evidence That Transient Changes in Sudomotor Output with Cold and Warm Fluid Ingestion Are Independently Modulated by Abdominal, but Not Oral Thermoreceptors," *Journal of Applied Physiology* 116, no. 8 (2014).

149 *perception is reality:* P. C. Castle et al., "Deception of Ambient and Body Core Temperature Improves Self Paced Cycling in Hot, Humid Conditions," *European Journal of Applied Physiology* 112, no. 1 (2012).

149 *your pace is slower* right from the start: R. Tucker et al., "Impaired Exercise Performance in the Heat Is Associated with an Anticipatory Reduction in Skeletal Muscle Recruitment," *Pflügers Archiv* 448, no. 4 (2004).

150 *researchers at France's National Sport Institute:* A. Marc et al., "Marathon Progress: Demography, Morphology and Environment," *Journal of Sports Sciences* 32, no. 6 (2014).

150 *bigger and taller runners at a subtle disadvantage:* "Advantages of Smaller Body Mass During Distance Running in Warm, Humid Environments," *Pflügers Archiv* 441, nos. 2–3 (2000).

150 *50 of the 58 heatstroke deaths:* A. J. Grundstein et al., "A Retrospective Analysis of American Football Hyperthermia Deaths in the United States," *International Journal of Biometeorology* 56, no. 1 (2012).

151 *Stephen Cheung:* Stephen Cheung and Tom McLellan, "Heat Acclimation, Aerobic Fitness, and Hydration Effects on Tolerance During Uncompensable Heat Stress," *Journal of Applied Physiology* 84, no. 5 (1998); P. J. Wallace et al., "Effects of Motivational

Self-Talk on Endurance and Cognitive Performance in the Heat," *Medicine & Science in Sports & Exercise* 49, no. 1 (2017).

152 *a revised definition of heatstroke:* Abderrezak Bouchama and James Knochel, "Heat Stroke," *New England Journal of Medicine* 346, no. 25 (2002).

152 *factors that nudge your heatstroke risk upward:* "Heat Stroke: Role of the Systemic Inflammatory Response," *Journal of Applied Physiology* 109, no. 6 (2010).

152 *British cyclist Tom Simpson:* William Fotheringham, *Put Me Back on My Bike* (London: Yellow Jersey Press, 2002).

153 *"so doped that he did not know . . ."*: J. L Manning, *Daily Mail*, July 31, 1967, as quoted by the Australian Associated Press in the *Age,* August 2, 1967.

153 *Eric Newsholme:* Lindy Castell, "Obituary for Professor Eric Arthur Newsholme, MA, Dsc, (PhD, ScD Camb)," BJSM Blog, April 7, 2011; Bart Roelands and Romain Meeusen, "Alterations in Central Fatigue by Pharmacological Manipulations of Neurotransmitters in Normal and High Ambient Temperature," *Sports Medicine* 40, no. 3 (2010).

154 *"Their 'safety brake' didn't work,"*: Romain Meeusen at the Nestlé Nutrition Institute Sport Nutrition Conference, Canberra, Australia, 2010.

154 *Gilpin's Adderall use:* Andrew Wolfson, "PRP Player Who Died Wasn't Dehydrated, Experts Say," *Louisville Courier-Journal,* March 8, 2009.

154 *heat-related football deaths tripled:* Grundstein, "A Retrospective Analysis"; Samuel Zuvekas and Benedetto Vitiello, "Stimulant Medication Use among U.S. Children: A Twelve-Year Perspective," *American Journal of Psychiatry* 169, no. 2 (2012).

154 *"I think you can almost take judicial notice . . ."*: As quoted in Lake.

CHAPTER 9: THIRST

157 *Pablo Valencia and Jesus Rios:* W. J. McGee, "Desert Thirst in Disease," *Interstate Medical Journal* 13 (1906): 1–23, reprinted in *Journal of the Southwest* 30, no. 2 (1988), along with commentary, Bill Broyles, "W J McGee's 'Desert Thirst as Disease.'" The case is discussed in Tim Noakes, *Waterlogged: The Serious Problem of Overhydration in Endurance Sports* (Champaign, IL: Human Kinetics, 2012).

157 *body is about 50 to 70 percent water:* Robert Kenefick et al., "Dehydration and Rehydration," in *Wilderness Medicine*, ed. Paul Auerbach (Philadelphia: Mosby Elsevier, 2011); Samuel Cheuvront et al., "Physiologic Basis for Understanding Quantitative Dehydration Assessment," *American Journal of Clinical Nutrition* 97, no. 3 (2013).

159 *the case of Andreas Mihavecz:* "Beamte vergaßen Häftling in der Zelle: Verurteilt," *Hamburger Abendblatt,* November 6, 1979; Guinness World Records, 2003.

160 *"Don't get in the habit . . ."*: Quoted in Tim Noakes, "Hyperthermia, Hypothermia and Problems of Hydration," in *Endurance in Sport*, ed. R. J. Shephard and P.-O. Astrand (Oxford: Blackwell, 2000).

160 *Amby Burfoot ran the Boston Marathon:* Amby Burfoot, "Running Scared," *Runner's World,* May 2008.

160 *"my football players do not wee wee . . ."*: Transcript, Dr. James Robert Cade, Oral History Interview with Samuel Procter, April 22, 1996, Samuel Proctor Oral History Program Collection, University of Florida; Richard Burnett, "Gatorade Inventor: My Success Based on Luck and Sweat," *Orlando Sentinel,* April 16, 1994.

161 *Gatorade-sponsored:* Darren Rovell, *First in Thirst: How Gatorade Turned the Science of Sweat into a Cultural Phenomenon* (New York: American Management Association, 2005).

161 *"replace all the water lost through sweating . . .":* V.A. Convertino et al., "American College of Sports Medicine Position Stand. Exercise and Fluid Replacement," *Medicine & Science in Sports & Exercise* 28, no. 1 (1996).

161 *death of twenty-eight-year-old Cynthia Lucero:* Noakes, *Waterlogged.*

161 *U.S.A. Track and Field rewrote their guidelines:* Gina Kolata, "New Advice to Runners: Don't Drink the Water," *New York Times,* May 6, 2003.

162 *"voluntary dehydration":* A. Rothstein et al., "Voluntary Dehydration," in *Physiology of Man in the Desert,* ed. E. F. Adolph (New York: Hafner, 1948).

162 *link dehydration more specifically with overheating:* C. H. Wyndham and N. B. Strydom, "The Danger of an Inadequate Water Intake During Marathon Running," *South African Medical Journal* 43, no. 29 (1969); D. L. Costill et al., "Fluid Ingestion During Distance Running," *Archives of Environmental Health* 21, no. 4 (1970).

163 *U.S. Army study in 1966:* E. N. Craig and E. G. Cummings, "Dehydration and Muscular Work," *Journal of Applied Physiology* 21, no. 2 (1966).

163 *recent accusations:* David Epstein, "Off Track: Former Team Members Accuse Famed Coach Alberto Salazar of Breaking Drug Rules," ProPublica, June 3, 2015.

163 *"You will never be broken again.":* Alberto Salazar and John Brant, *14 Minutes: A Running Legend's Life and Death and Life* (Emmaus, PA: Rodale, 2013).

164 *"Duel in the Sun.":* John Brant, *Duel in the Sun: Alberto Salazar, Dick Beardsley, and America's Greatest Marathon* (Emmaus, PA: Rodale, 2006). The label was first applied to the race by Neil Amdur in the first sentence of his article for the *New York Times,* "Salazar Wins Fastest Boston Marathon," April 20, 1982.

165 *an unusually high three liters of sweat per hour:* L. E. Armstrong et al., "Preparing Alberto Salazar for the Heat of the 1984 Olympic Marathon," *Physician and Sportsmedicine* 14, no. 3 (1986).

165 *body temperature was measured as 88 degrees:* Thomas Boswell, "Salazar Sets Record in Boston Marathon," *Washington Post,* April 20, 1982.

165 *William Castelli:* As quoted in Heyward Nash, "Treating Thermal Injury: Disagreement Heats Up," *Physician and Sportsmedicine* 13, no. 7 (1985).

166 *a guest on an NPR affiliate: The Colin McEnroe Show,* WNPR, May 26, 2016. Audio available at http://wnpr.org/post/how-much-water-do-you-need.

167 *Gebrselassie sweats at a prodigious rate:* Lukas Beis et al., "Drinking Behaviors of Elite Male Runners During Marathon Competition," *Clinical Journal of Sports Medicine* 22, no. 3 (2012).

168 *Mont Saint-Michel Marathon:* Hassane Zouhal et al., "Inverse Relationship Between Percentage Body Weight Change and Finishing Time in 643 Forty-Two-Kilometre Marathon Runners," *British Journal of Sports Medicine* 45, no. 14 (2011).

168 *athletes needing assistance or even collapsing after the finish of a long race:* Cameron Anley, "A Comparison of Two Treatment Protocols in the Management of Exercise-Associated Postural Hypotension: A Randomised Clinical Trial," *British Journal of Sports Medicine* 45 (2010): 1113–18.

169 *a distinction between thirst . . . and dehydration:* M. N. Sawka and T. D. Noakes, "Does Hydration Impair Exercise Performance?," *Medicine & Science in Sports & Exercise* 39, no. 8 (2007).

170 *your body monitors "plasma osmolality,":* Cheuvront, "Physiologic Basis."

170 *South African Special Forces soldiers:* Heinrich Nolte et al., "Trained Humans

Can Exercise Safely in Extreme Dry Heat When Drinking Water Ad Libitum," *Journal of Sports Sciences* 29, no. 12 (2011).

170 *!Xo San Bushman hunter Karoha Langwane:* Cited in Nolte, "Trained Humans."
171 *a marathoner could conceivably lose 1 to 3 percent:* R. J. Maughan et al., "Errors in the Estimation of Hydration Status from Changes in Body Mass," *Journal of Sports Sciences* 25, no. 7 (2007); N. Tam et al., "Changes in Total Body Water Content During Running Races of 21.1 km and 56 km in Athletes Drinking Ad Libitum," *Clinical Journal of Sports Medicine* 21, no. 3 (2011).
172 *data from the Western States:* Martin Hoffman et al., "Don't Lose More than 2% of Body Mass During Ultra-Endurance Running. Really?" *International Journal of Sports Physiology and Performance* 12, no. S1 (2017).
172 *a 2009 study at Noakes's lab:* J. P. Dugas et al., "Rates of Fluid Ingestion Alter Pacing but Not Thermoregulatory Responses During Prolonged Exercise in Hot and Humid Conditions with Appropriate Convective Cooling," *European Journal of Applied Physiology* 105, no. 1 (2009).
173 *"very unlikely to impair . . .":* E. D. Goulet, "Effect of Exercise-Induced Dehydration on Endurance Performance: Evaluating the Impact of Exercise Protocols on Outcomes Using a Meta-Analytic Procedure," *British Journal of Sports Medicine* 47, no. 11 (2013).
173 *hydrating a group of cyclists intravenously:* S. S. Cheung et al., "Separate and Combined Effects of Dehydration and Thirst Sensation on Exercise Performance in the Heat," *Scandinavian Journal of Medicine & Science in Sports* 25 (2015): 104–11.
173 *famous 1997 study at Yale:* M. Kathleen Figaro and Gary W. Mack, "Regulation of Fluid Intake in Dehydrated Humans: Role of Oropharyngeal Stimulation," *American Journal of Physiology* 272, no. 41 (1997).
174 *swallowing small mouthfuls of water:* G. Arnaoutis et al., "Water ingestion improves performance compared with mouth rinse in dehydrated subjects," *Medicine & Science in Sports & Exercise* 44, no. 1 (2012).
175 *"Anyone who has worked in the field . . .":* Alex Hutchinson, "How Much Water Should You Drink? Research Is Changing What We Know About Our Fluid Needs," *Globe and Mail,* May 31, 2015.
175 *During his 2007 world record race:* Alex Hutchinson, "Haile Gebrselassie's World Record Marathon Fueling Plan," *Runner's World,* November 8, 2013.
176 *staying hydrated is actually* bad: Gregor Brown, "'Dehydration Could Make You Climb Faster' Says Top Team Medical Consultant," *Cycling Weekly,* December 5, 2016.

CHAPTER 10: FUEL

177 *". . . where things got weird,":* Alex Hutchinson, "The Latest on Low-Carb, High-Fat Diets," *Outside,* March 9, 2016; Alex Hutchinson, "Canadian Race Walker Evan Dunfee Taking Part in Study on High-Fat Diets," *Globe and Mail,* January 26, 2017.
178 *"For 33 years I followed . . .":* Joe Friel, *Fast After 50* (Boulder, CO: VeloPress, 2015).
178 *code-named "Supernova.":* Louise Burke et al., "Low Carbohydrate, High Fat Diet Impairs Exercise Economy and Negates the Performance Benefit from Intensified Training in Elite Race Walkers," *Journal of Physiology* 595, no. 9 (2017).
179 *Kieran Doherty:* Jessica Hamzelou, "Maxed Out: How Long Could You Survive Without Food or Drink?," *New Scientist,* April 14, 2010.

179 *the case of A.B.:* W. K. Stewart and Laura W. Fleming, "Features of a Successful Therapeutic Fast of 382 Days' Duration," *Postgraduate Medical Journal* 49 (1973): 203–9.

180 *skipping breakfast:* D. J. Clayton et al., "Effect of Breakfast Omission on Energy Intake and Evening Exercise Performance," *Medicine & Science in Sports & Exercise* 47, no. 12 (2015).

180 *researchers at the University of Minnesota:* Tucker, *The Great Starvation Experiment.*

180 *protein can contribute up to 10 percent:* Hiroyuki Kato et al., "Protein Requirements Are Elevated in Endurance Athletes After Exercise as Determined by the Indicator Amino Acid Oxidation Method," *PLoS One* 11, no. 6 (2016).

180 *Early experiments in the first half:* Andrew Coggan, "Metabolic Systems: Substrate Utilization," in *History of Exercise Physiology,* ed. Tipton.

181 *97 percent carbohydrate fuel:* M. J. O'Brien et al., "Carbohydrate Dependence During Marathon Running," *Medicine & Science in Sports & Exercise* 25, no. 9 (1993).

181 *Bergström pioneered:* Jonas Bergström and Eric Hultman, "Muscle Glycogen after Exercise: an Enhancing Factor localized to the Muscle Cells in Man," *Nature* 210, no. 5033 (1966); see also John Hawley et al., "Exercise Metabolism: Historical Perspective," *Cell Metabolism* 22, no. 1 (2015).

182 *can store 400 or 500 calories:* Benjamin Rapoport, "Metabolic Factors Limiting Performance in Marathon Runners," *PLoS Computational Biology* 6, no. 10 (2010).

182 *study found that Kenyan runners:* "Food and Macronutrient Intake of Elite Kenyan Distance Runners," *International Journal of Sport Nutrition and Exercise Metabolism* 14, no. 6 (2005).

182 *Ethiopians; a similar study:* Lukas Beis et al., "Food and Macronutrient Intake of Elite Ethiopian Distance Runners," *Journal of the International Society of Sports Nutrition* 8, no. 7 (2011).

183 *Frederick Schwatka and his companions:* William Gilder, *Schwatka's Search: Sledging in the Arctic in Quest of the Franklin Records,* 1881; Ronald Savitt, "Frederick Schwatka and the Search for the Franklin Expedition Records, 1878–1880," *Polar Record* 44, no. 230 (2008).

183 *"a Chinese gong . . .":* Bill Bryson, *In a Sunburned Country* (New York: Random House, 2001).

184 *"And he possesses a very important adjunct, . . .":* Gilder, *Schwatka's Search.*

184 *"When first thrown wholly . . .":* F. Schwatka, *The Long Arctic Search,* ed. E. Stackpole, reprinted 1965, quoted in Stephen Phinney, "Ketogenic Diets and Physical Performance," *Nutrition & Metabolism* 1, no. 2 (2004).

184 *Vilhjalmur Stefansson, reached similar conclusions:* Vilhjalmur Stefansson, "Adventures in Diet (Part II)," *Harper's Magazine,* December 1935.

185 *published in 1930 in the Journal of Biological Chemistry:* Walter S. McClellan and Eugene F. Du Bois, "Prolonged Meat Diets with a Study of Kidney Function and Ketosis," *Journal of Biological Chemistry* 87 (1930): 651–68.

185 *published in 1945 in the journal War Medicine:* R. M. Kark, "Defects of Pemmican as an Emergency Ration for Infantry Troops," June 1945, quotation from a summary in *Nutrition Reviews,* October 1945.

186 *Stephen Phinney pointed out in 1983:* S. D. Phinney et al., "The Human Metabolic Response to Chronic Ketosis Without Caloric Restriction: Preservation of Submax-

imal Exercise Capability with Reduced Carbohydrate Oxidation," *Metabolism* 32, no. 8 (1983).

186 *takes around 3,000 calories:* Rapoport, "Metabolic Factors."

186 *at least 30,000:* Jeff Volek et al., "Rethinking Fat as a Fuel for Endurance Exercise," *European Journal of Sport Science* 15, no. 1 (2014).

187 *a definitive 2005 study at the University of Cape Town:* L. Havemann et al., "Fat Adaptation Followed by Carbohydrate Loading Compromises High-Intensity Sprint Performance," *Journal of Applied Physiology* 100, no. 1 (2006); L. M. Burke and B. Kiens, "'Fat Adaptation' for Athletic Performance: The Nail in the Coffin?," *Journal of Applied Physiology* 100, no. 1 (2006); T. Stellingwerff et al., "Decreased PDH Activation and Glycogenolysis During Exercise Following Fat Adaptation with Carbohydrate Restoration," *American Journal of Physiology–Endocrinology and Metabolism* 290, no. 2 (2006).

188 *combine two different types of carbohydrate:* R. L. Jentjens et al., "Oxidation of Combined Ingestion of Glucose and Fructose During Exercise," *Journal of Applied Physiology* 696, no. 4 (2004).

189 *don't just act as energy reservoirs:* "Muscle glycogen stores and fatigue," N. Ørtenblad et al., *Journal of Physiology*, 2013, 591(18).

189 *as little as half an hour:* Ian Rollo et al., "The Influence of Carbohydrate Mouth Rinse on Self-Selected Speeds During a 30-min Treadmill Run," *International Journal of Sport Nutrition and Exercise Metabolism* 18 (2008): 585–600.

190 *they asked the cyclists to swish:* J. M. Carter et al., "The Effect of Carbohydrate Mouth Rinse on 1-h Cycle Time Trial Performance," *Medicine & Science in Sports & Exercise* 36, no. 12 (2004).

190 *used functional magnetic resonance imaging:* E. S. Chambers et al., "Carbohydrate Sensing in the Human Mouth: Effects on Exercise Performance and Brain Activity," *Journal of Physiology* 587, no. 8 (2009).

190 *Brazilian researchers had cyclists:* T. Ataide-Silva et al., "CHO Mouth Rinse Ameliorates Neuromuscular Response with Lower Endogenous CHO Stores," *Medicine & Science in Sports & Exercise* 48, no. 9 (2016).

191 Men's Journal *ran a much-circulated article:* Dorsey Kindler, "Paleo's Latest Converts," June 18, 2013.

192 *fat-adapted runners were able to burn fat:* J. S. Volek et al., "Metabolic Characteristics of Keto-Adapted Ultra-Endurance Runners," *Metabolism* 65, no. 3 (2016).

192 *keep overall carbohydrate intake low:* Alex Hutchinson, "The High-Fat Diet for Runners," *Outside,* November 2014.

192 *diet followed by two-time Olympic triathlon medalist Simon Whitfield:* "Whitfield: What Do You Eat?," SimonWhitfield.com, August 1, 2008, https://simonwhitfield.blogspot.ca/2008/08/glo.html.

194 *To prove the cyclists wrong:* Louise Burke, Ben Desbrow, and Lawrence Spriet, *Caffeine and Sports Performance* (Champaign, IL: Human Kinetics, 2013).

194 *The Supernova results:* Burke, "Low Carbohydrate."

196 *a pair of studies in 2016 using a protocol dubbed "sleep low,":* L. A. Marquet et al., "Enhanced Endurance Performance by Periodization of Carbohydrate Intake: 'Sleep Low' Strategy," *Medicine & Science in Sports & Exercise* 48, no. 4 (2016); L. A. Marquet et al., "Periodization of Carbohydrate Intake: Short-Term Effect on Performance," *Nutrients* 8, no. 12 (2016).

197 *mountain guide Adrian Ballinger:* Marissa Stephenson, "How Adrian Ballinger Summited Everest Without Oxygen," *Men's Journal,* May 27, 2017; Kyle McCall, "Everest No Filter: The Second Ascent," *Strava Stories,* June 7, 2017.

199 *"The cramps were fierce . . .":* "Have At It," Mark Twight, press release issued after climbing Slovak Direct in 2000, https://www.marktwight.com/blogs/discourse/84295748 -have-at-it.

TWO HOURS: MARCH 6, 2017

202 *Tesla pace car:* Alex Hutchinson, "Did the Tesla Pace Car Aid Eliud Kipchoge's 2:00:25 Marathon?," *Runner's World,* May 24, 2017.

203 *". . . two painful seconds . . .":* Roger Bannister, *The Four-Minute Mile* (New York: Dodd, Mead, 1955).

204 *some expedition members felt its use was unsporting:* Reinhold Messner, *Everest: Expedition to the Ultimate* (New York: Oxford University Press, 1979).

204 *a grainy CT scan:* Jeré Longman, "Do Nike's New Shoes Give Runners an Unfair Advantage?," *New York Times,* March 8, 2017.

206 *"The verdict was that I'm ready . . .":* Peter Njenga, "Marathon King on a Mission to Break 'Impossible' Record," *Daily Nation,* February 12, 2017.

207 *"The difference only is thinking,":* "Kenyan Star Prepares 'Crazy' Sub-2 Marathon Bid," Agence France-Presse, April 3, 2017.

CHAPTER 11: TRAINING THE BRAIN

210 *collaborators such as Alan St. Clair Gibson:* Alan St. Clair Gibson et al., "The Conscious Perception of the Sensation of Fatigue," *Sports Medicine* 33, no. 3 (2003).

210 *Ross Tucker, published a paper:* R. Tucker, "The Anticipatory Regulation of Performance: The Physiological Basis for Pacing Strategies and the Development of a Perception-Based Model for Exercise Performance," *British Journal of Sports Medicine* 43, no. 6 (2009).

211 *the brain's* outgoing *signals:* This is a fascinating physiological question, but one that ends up making little practical difference to the research discussed in the book. Exercising with tired muscles may be challenging because the muscles send distress signals back to the brain, or it may be challenging because the brain has to send stronger outgoing signals to get the same muscle response. The net result, in most contexts, is the same. My guess is that there's a little bit of both going on. For more, see M. Amann and N. H. Secher, "Point: Afferent feedback from fatigued locomotor muscles is an important determinant of endurance exercise performance," *Journal of Applied Physiology* 108, no. 2 (2009); Helma de Morree and Samuele Marcora, "Psychobiology of Perceived Effort During Physical Tasks," in *Handbook of Biobehavioral Approaches to Self-Regulation* (New York: Springer, 2015).

212 *famous Emo Phillips joke:* Emo Phillips, "The Best God Joke Ever—and It's Mine!," *Guardian,* September 29, 2005.

213 *On my first day at the University of Kent's:* The visit and my experiences with brain endurance training were first described in "How to Build Mental Muscle," *Runner's World,* October 2013.

213 *a new effort-based protocol:* A. R. Mauger and N. Sculthorpe, "A New VO_2-max Protocol Allowing Self-Pacing in Maximal Incremental Exercise," *British Journal of Sports Medicine* 46, no. 1 (2012).

214 *another study, from Noakes's group:* F. G. Beltrami et al., "Conventional Testing Methods Produce Submaximal Values of Maximum Oxygen Consumption," *British Journal of Sports Medicine* 46, no. 1 (2012).

216 *a particularly graphic illustration of its importance:* C. R. Wagstaff, "Emotion Regulation and Sport Performance," *Journal of Sport and Exercise Psychology* 36, no. 4 (2014).

221 *Staiano and Marcora presented recently declassified results:* Walter Staiano et al., "A Randomized Controlled Trial of Brain Endurance Training (BET) to Reduce Fatigue During Endurance Exercise," *Medicine & Science in Sports & Exercise* 47, no. 5S (2015).

221 *a 2016 analysis of virtually every brain-training study:* Daniel Simons et al., "Do 'Brain-Training' Programs Work?," *Psychological Science in the Public Interest* 17, no. 3 (2016).

222 *"'This is not happening! Why now?'":* I first wrote about Isaković, and Paulus's research, in "Cracking the Athlete's Brain," *Outside,* February 2014.

225 *followed eight Marine infantry platoons:* L. Haase et al., "Mindfulness-Based Training Attenuates Insula Response to an Aversive Interoceptive Challenge," *Social Cognitive and Affective Neuroscience* 11, no. 1 (2016).

225 *hardened Navy SEALs and elite adventure racers:* M. P. Paulus et al., "Subjecting Elite Athletes to Inspiratory Breathing Load Reveals Behavioral and Neural Signatures of Optimal Performers in Extreme Environments," *PLoS One* 7, no. 1 (2012).

226 *athletes from the U.S. Olympic BMX racing team:* L. Haase, "A Pilot Study Investigating Changes in Neural Processing After Mindfulness Training in Elite Athletes," *Frontiers in Behavioral Neuroscience* 9, no. 229 (2015); see also Alex Hutchinson, "Can Mindfulness Training Make You a Better Athlete?," *Outside,* September 15, 2015.

226 *"Their body language is calmer . . .":* quoted in Christina Johnson, "Mindfulness Training Program May Help Olympic Athletes Reach Peak Performance," UC San Diego News Center, June 5, 2014.

CHAPTER 12: ZAPPING THE BRAIN

229 *A sharp bang:* I wrote about Red Bull's Project Endurance in "Your Body on Brain Doping," *Outside,* August 2, 2014.

230 *Scribonius Largus:* C. I. Sarmiento et al., "Brief History of Transcranial Direct Current Stimulation (tDCS): From Electric Fishes to Microcontrollers," *Psychological Medicine* 46, no. 3259 (2016).

231 *freshly decapitated criminals:* André Parent, "Giovanni Aldini: From Animal Electricity to Human Brain Stimulation," *Canadian Journal of Neurological Sciences* 31 (2004): 576–84.

232 *tango dancing:* D. Kaski et al., "Applying Anodal tDCS During Tango Dancing in a Patient with Parkinson's Disease," *Neuroscience Letters* 568 (2014): 39–43.

232 *ability to spot snipers:* Vincent Clark et al., "TDCS Guided Using fMRI Significantly Accelerates Learning to Identify Concealed Objects," *NeuroImage* 59, no. 1 (2012).

232 *"a sea of bullshit . . .":* Emily Underwood, "Cadaver Study Casts Doubts on How Zapping Brain May Boost Mood, Relieve Pain," *Science,* April 20, 2016.

233 *tested on handgrip strength:* L. Hilty et al., "Limitation of Physical Performance in a Muscle Fatiguing Handgrip Exercise Is Mediated by Thalamo-Insular Activity," *Human Brain Mapping* 32, no. 12 (2011).

234 *In the EEG study:* "Fatigue-Induced Increase in Intracortical Communication

Between Mid/Anterior Insular and Motor Cortex During Cycling Exercise," *European Journal of Neuroscience* 34, no. 12 (2011).

235 *published four years earlier by Alberto Priori:* F. Cogiamanian et al., "Improved Isometric Force Endurance After Transcranial Direct Current Stimulation over the Human Motor Cortical Areas," *European Journal of Neuroscience* 26, no. 1 (2007).

235 *brain stimulation test on ten national-class cyclists:* Alexandre Okano et al., "Brain Stimulation Modulates the Autonomic Nervous System, Rating of Perceived Exertion and Performance During Maximal Exercise," *British Journal of Sports Medicine* 49, no. 18 (2015).

236 *including the prefrontal cortex:* C. V. Robertson and F. E. Marino, "A Role for the Prefrontal Cortex in Exercise Tolerance and Termination," *Journal of Applied Physiology* 120, no. 4 (2016).

238 *James Michael McAdoo, a power forward:* Alex Hutchinson, "For the Golden State Warriors, Brain Zapping Could Provide an Edge," *New Yorker,* June 15, 2016.

239 *reviewed the existing literature on how tDCS:* Luca Angius et al., "The Ergogenic Effects of Transcranial Direct Current Stimulation on Exercise Performance," *Frontiers in Physiology,* February 14, 2017.

241 *apparently safe:* A. Antal et al., "Low Intensity Transcranial Electric Stimulation: Safety, Ethical, Legal Regulatory and Application guidelines," *Clinical Neurophysiology,* June 19, 2017.

242 *electrode on the shoulder:* L. Angius et al., "Transcranial Direct Current Stimulation Improves Isometric Time to Exhaustion of the Knee Extensors," *Neuroscience* 339 (2016): 363–75; L. Angius et al., "Transcranial direct current stimulation improves cycling performance in healthy individuals," *Proceedings of The Physiological Society* 35, no. C03.

CHAPTER 13: BELIEF

246 *Reid Coolsaet was wide awake:* I wrote about Coolsaet's marathon in "The Race Against Time," *Walrus,* July/August 2012.

248 *a manual-laborer-turned-runner named Joseph Nderitu:* Alex Hutchinson, "Any Race, Every Weekend," Ottawa Citizen, May 28, 2006.

247 *he noticed that Kenyan and Western runners had markedly different mentalities:* "Trampled Under Foot," www.reidcoolsaet.com, February 9, 2013.

250 *Shona Halson and David Martin:* Shona Halson and David Martin, "Lying to Win—Placebos and Sport Science," *International Journal of Sports Physiology and Performance* 8 (2013): 597–99.

251 *purported benefits of a post-workout ice bath:* J. Leeder, "Cold Water Immersion and Recovery from Strenuous Exercise: A Meta-Analysis," *British Journal of Sports Medicine* 46, no. 4 (2012).

251 *a "placebo-controlled" ice bath:* J. R. Broatch et al., "Postexercise Cold Water Immersion Benefits Are Not Greater than the Placebo Effect," *Medicine & Science in Sports & Exercise* 46, no. 11 (2014).

252 *paradigm-altering demonstration:* J. D. Levine et al., "The Mechanism of Placebo Analgesia," *Lancet* 2, no. 8091 (1978).

253 *placebo-driven expectations:* Sumathi Reddy, "Why Placebos Really Work: The Latest Science," *Wall Street Journal,* July 18, 2016.

253 *treat irritable bowel syndrome:* Kathryn Hall et al., "Catechol-O-Methyltrans-

ferase val158met Polymorphism Predicts Placebo Effect in Irritable Bowel Syndrome," *PLoS One* 7, no. 10 (2012).

253 *cyclists rode 1.3 percent faster:* C. J. Beedie et al., "Placebo Effects of Caffeine on Cycling Performance," *Medicine & Science in Sports & Exercise* 38, no. 12 (2006).

254 *whether lucky charms actually work:* L. Damisch et al., "Keep Your Fingers Crossed! How Superstition Improves Performance," *Psychological Science* 21, no. 7 (2010).

254 *Telling runners they look relaxed:* I. Stoate et al., "Enhanced Expectancies Improve Movement Efficiency in Runners," *Journal of Sports Sciences* 30, no. 8 (2012).

254 *rugby players a postgame debriefing:* B. T. Crewther and C. J. Cook, "Effects of Different Post-Match Recovery Interventions on Subsequent Athlete Hormonal State and Game Performance," *Physiology & Behavior* 106, no. 4 (2012).

254 *doing a good deed:* Kurt Gray, "Moral Transformation: Good and Evil Turn the Weak into the Mighty," *Social Psychological and Personality Science* 1, no. 3 (2010).

254 *fueled by "pure hate":* As articulated in a classic thread on the Letsrun.com message boards, "Running the 800 on Pure Hate," November 17, 2008.

255 *". . . best running workout you can do.":* Amby Burfoot, "Milkshakes, Mile Repeats, and Your Mind: A Delicious Combination," *Runner's World,* June 12, 2011.

255 *using various forms of deception:* E. L. Williams, "Deception Studies Manipulating Centrally Acting Performance Modifiers: A Review," *Medicine & Science in Sports & Exercise* 46, no. 7 (2014).

255 *Race against a two-percent-improved version:* G. P. Ducrocq et al., "Increased Fatigue Response to Augmented Deceptive Feedback During Cycling Time Trial," *Medicine & Science in Sports & Exercise* 49, no. 8 (2017).

256 *ready to run 2:05:* "You Were Springing Like a Gazelle," www.reidcoolsaet.com, January 27, 2012.

257 *Kentucky Derby and the Epsom Derby:* D. S. Gardner, "Historical Progression of Racing Performance in Thoroughbreds and Man," *Equine Veterinary Journal* 38, no. 6 (2006).

257 *justified beliefs and true beliefs:* Edmund Gettier, "Is Justified True Belief Knowledge?," *Analysis* 23, no. 6 (1963).

259 *Run a lot of miles:* Joyner sent me the haiku in an email on February 3, 2016, and has since been quoted on it elsewhere.

259 *Steve Magness has written:* "A Case for Running by Feel—Ditching Your GPS Because of Ecological Psychology," scienceofrunning.com, February 8, 2016.

260 *grueling sixty-mile overnight ultramarathon:* A. McCormick et al., "The Effects of Self-Talk on Performance in an Ultramarathon," presented at the Endurance Research Conference, University of Kent, September 2015.

TWO HOURS: MAY 6, 2017

266 *experimental Swedish sports drink:* Alex Hutchinson, "After a Near Sub-2 Marathon, What's Next?," *Runner's World,* May 6, 2017.

266 *external testing of the Vaporfly:* Hoogkamer, "New Running Shoe."

Index